I0481149

# Nurse Life

## An Unofficial Guide to Becoming a Nurse and Understanding the Nursing World

By: Brett Craigsly

# Brett Craigsly

Printed in the United States of America

First Printing, 2021

**ISBN:** 9798724069755

# Privacy and Educational Disclaimers:

Privacy laws are strict and unforgiving. As this can be considered a non-fiction informational book, I shared a few anecdotes and stories that will be of value in characterizing a working environment. These stories are intended solely for educational purposes. I have not disclosed the states or cities in which I lived or worked as a nurse. I have not disclosed the names of any healthcare organizations for whom I've worked. I have not disclosed the names or locations of any schools which I have attended for nursing or any other education.

Anecdotal stories may include the most basic of information, such as a gender and age, as it is necessary for the educational spirit of the narrative. No other personal or identifying patient information has been shared. Events described are common enough that an anecdote will not identify a single patient. I have not referenced any famous or well-known events in the country, which might help to identify a patient. There is not sufficient evidence to "triangulate" a patient based on multiple pieces of information.

No actual or perceived medical expertise or opinion in this reading should be taken as solid fact to be used in the treatment of any other patient. As you will read in my story, I haven't been working for about two years at the time I'm writing this, and so my advanced critical care knowledge and awareness of the healthcare industry may be slightly outdated. These things change constantly. I can't absolutely guarantee that every piece of medical knowledge is 100% accurate and up-to-date in the ever-evolving world of medicine. Some concepts may be dated.

This is not a text book, and I have not given full or

complete instruction on how to manage any given situation. That's what nursing school and clinical rotations will do for you. But I intended to at least give you a taste of what's to come. If your nursing text book, your nursing instructor, your boss, a physician, or even your own medical expertise is in conflict with anything I say, follow those directions, and leave me out of it.

Please also note that as I share stories, I am in no way laughing, joking, or otherwise telling the stories in a way that is intended to be funny, or overly shocking. These are not jokes. They were real people.

# Chapter 1: Introduction

I have been a nurse for about 12 years, although I have not worked in the last two of those years. I have lots of stories to tell and wisdom to share from my experiences. In addition to my goals and work in critical care, I had aspired to eventually teach in a nursing school. I never got the chance to do that. I learned so much over the years from those with more experience than myself. I believe that medical expertise comes not from a text book, but from real-life interactions and experiences. I was often asked how I became so good at starting IV's. The answer was that I had started thousands of IV's. That is not something you can learn from a book. It takes repetition. And nursing as a whole is no different. From every encounter with a patient, boss, peer, coworker, educator, or mentor over your career, you will gain new knowledge, insight, perspective, and experience. It will come in tiny increments, but it builds into expertise.

Considering I never got to try out teaching, I thought I would write a book that might help aspiring nurses learn something about their chosen field. Perhaps this can count as one of those "encounter" repetitions when you learn something new from someone who has "been there and done that." I hope I can help you in some way, even if you just learn one little detail. That will then be one little detail about which you will be wiser and more experienced when you begin your practice.

I want to start by clearly defining what this book is, and what it is not.

This book is meant to be enjoyable to read. It's not a text book. It's not a reference book. It's not an autobiography. It's not meant to glorify anything I've done, nor is it meant to appear as a memoir. It does not claim to have the full archive of wisdom and knowledge society has amassed over the millennia. It's just stories and information that <u>might</u> be helpful or enjoyable to a nurse, nursing student, or person who is considering nursing school. Your first priority in reading this book should be to enjoy it.

I like to think I am funny. I will try to be. I may fail. You can be the judge of that.

When I was planning for, and attending nursing school, I was like a sponge trying to soak up every ounce of knowledge I could. I was excited about the job I would do. Over the years I have been cornered by numerous individuals seeking to ask me questions about nursing, as they too aspire to join our ranks, are excited about the work they will do, and are like more sponges soaking up information.

If this is your disposition, and you are thirsty for knowledge, then I invite you to stand under me and let me wring my sponge of expertise and pour my knowledge and experience juices onto you. (Did that come out right? Ha!) And, one day, when you are the veteran hot-shot ICU nurse, and someone asks you the secret to your success, you will remember me and how I inspired you to achievements beyond your wildest dreams. Or, probably not. Either way is fine.

Nursing is an exciting and tremendously fulfilling line of work, one in which many lives are touched, and a genuine difference can be made. However, television and movies generally fail to offer a realistic grasp of the nursing experience. Just as real lawyers hate legal dramas, and police officers hate crime dramas, I can't stand to watch medical shows or movies. I find myself pointing out every technical flaw, misrepresentation, and inaccuracy along the way.

Ultimately, it's important to understand that hospital life is very different from how it looks on television. I've come to believe that it's imperative for aspiring nursing

4

students to truly understand what is ahead if they choose this career path.

Before I get into the meat of my experiences in nursing, I want to revisit the disclaimer that this book represents my experience, and mine alone. I've worked in a variety of different settings, but there are many areas in which I have no knowledge or experience. If I get into a subject that I know very little about, I will tell you. I do not claim to be all-knowing about every aspect of nursing, nor do I even claim to be a well-rounded expert in any one area. My experiences might fairly represent the average nurse who spends time in some of the more common settings. Some (or many) other nurses may disagree with my particular assessments of the profession, based on their own experiences in other facilities or settings. If you were to line up 50,000 nurses and ask them each individually about their opinions and experiences in nursing, you would likely get 50,000 different and unique answers. My single experience and opinion is only one of a limitless number of possibilities.

I will discuss some anecdotes of encounters with patients and staff, and share some of the heroics and excitement, along with the challenges and frustrations

Additionally, it is important for you to know what sort of content will be in this book. This will be a full-throttle uncensored and graphic description of the nursing experience. There may even be some PG-13 language. It is not for those with a weak stomach. I will not hold back in discussing the various aspects of caring for the human body, and I will include some realistic descriptions of the various anatomical structures, bodily functions, organs, fluids, waste products, drainage, excretions, secretions, growths, amputations, sights, smells, textures, sounds, and how the nurse interacts with them.

Once more, my experiences and opinions are neither all-inclusive nor exhaustive. Any technical medical information shared should always be confirmed through a thorough nursing assessment, and/or through a physician before you take action. I only ask that you read with an open mind, and I certainly encourage you to consider your own perspective and opinions in approaching the content of the reading. If you disagree with me, that is perfectly fine and acceptable. I'm just one man with one story. I hope to entertain you with the reading. I hope to make you laugh a few times. I hope to dismiss any myths or inaccurate preconceived notions. I hope that my story can help others who wish to follow in my footsteps. And maybe I can slip a little inspiration in too.

# Chapter 2:    My Story

Again, this book is not about me, but my story might offer a reasonable description of what one might expect.

I am a male, which has become quite common in nursing. We male nurses have a sort of funny saying when someone refers to our being a "male nurse." We respond with, "no, I take care of females too." That is an old and worn out joke, that you have probably heard by now. It's only mildly amusing, but calls out a continued social stigma attached with various career choices.    People tend to have paired specific gender identities with different jobs, and being a male nurse is one that some people question. Asking a male why he became a nurse often has a different approach than when asking a female, as if there's some extra motivation or factors that would make a man want to do a "woman's job."  Also, some might even attempt to question the sexual orientation of a man who wants to be a nurse, as if they think it takes a gay man to want to do a "woman's job." But, nursing is not a "woman's job," and we may dismiss that viewpoint.

The reality of nursing is quite different. The nursing workforce is indeed dominated by females, but males are becoming less a minority, and gaining traction as a fixture in the profession. During my decade of experience, I worked with people from every imaginable nationality, males and females, homosexual men and women, and on a couple of occasions trans-gender individuals. They were all equally capable and competent as nursing professionals, and I enjoyed working with all of them.   As a male, I hope to also provide some comfort to those other men out there who are considering being a nurse, but fear the potential social ramifications. It's perfectly okay to be a male nurse. I promise. (Plus you're surrounded by lots of pretty female nurses all day at work, which is awesome!)

I began my nursing career when I was in my late 20's. At the time of this writing, I'm now in my early 40's. I'm married with two children, and had otherwise enjoyed a seemingly "normal" existence, before some major life events (unrelated to my career as a nurse) sort of turned things upside down.

My general background was in business, however I became involved in both paid and volunteer firefighting, and emergency medical services work when I was in my mid-20's. I had attended training, and obtained the basic certifications needed for these activities. After a few years of this sort of exposure to healthcare, responding to medical calls and car accidents as a firefighter and EMT, I made a decision to change my trajectory in life.

I had immediately fallen in love with, and developed a passion for helping people and working in medical emergencies. It brought action and excitement, the type of thrill that couldn't be matched by any other extracurricular activity outside of my 8-5 Monday-Friday job. I also enjoyed the fact that my job would no longer focus on just money... who owes the company money, who the company owes money to, what happens with other people's money, if there is enough money, how the company can make more money, etc...

As a nurse, my job would revolve around caring for another person and their medical needs. Worrying about their insurance or financial status or ability to pay was somebody else's problem. I only focused on the skill of providing excellent and expert medical care.

After examining the career trajectory for firefighting, EMS, and nursing, I quickly discovered that nursing would offer the best earning potential, career and work diversity, and education and growth potential. I exited my business-style job, and applied to nursing school. While waiting to get into nursing school, and then also while in school, I worked as a certified nursing assistant (CNA) in a hospital. This job paid very little, and was back-breaking, but offered valuable hands-on experience. Between my wife's job and my CNA job, and with student loans, we made ends meet

I eventually began a one-year program to be a licensed practical nurse (LPN) or licensed vocational nurse (LVN), basically the same thing, just different name depending on what state you're in. I worked weekend nights at the local hospital as a CNA, and attended school basically 8 a.m. to 5 p.m. Monday through Thursday.

Once I was licensed as a LPN/LVN, I worked in a nursing home, hospital, and for a home health agency. Over the next couple of years I completed an associate's degree in nursing, along with becoming licensed as a registered nurse (RN). I continued with the same sort of work I had already been doing as an LPN, but now as an RN, and with a higher scope of practice, and while taking on leadership duties. I later completed a bachelor's of science degree in nursing (BSN). I began work on a master's degree in nursing, but did not finish.

I worked in a nursing home for about a year as my first job out of LPN school. I then worked about a year on a Med/Surg unit in a hospital. I spent about a year in the emergency department of the same hospital, and meanwhile completed my RN during this period. I then did another year of Med/Surg as an RN. I then transferred to an intermediate care unit for a couple of years, and finally the ICU, where I eventually reached my goal of being a charge nurse in a critical care unit. The span lasted about 10 years. My job in the ICU was the best, most enjoyable, most fulfilling, and most rewarding job I have ever had.

A complex and difficult set of life circumstances

(unrelated to nursing) led to me stopping my work. I won't tell that story. It doesn't matter in the context of this book. I don't know when or if I will return to work. Time will tell.

I love being a nurse, and miss my job terribly. I was among the very few people on this planet who could say, "I have the coolest job in the world." Once I was in nursing, I never considered, or had any desire to leave. I couldn't imagine doing anything different.

Many nursing students have a "dream" and "passion" for wanting to be a nurse, and some of them will fulfill this hope. Many will love their new life as a nurse. I did. Many others may find the job isn't what they thought it was going to be. Many may find they can't stand it once they start doing it for real. Nursing is not for everyone. It takes a special kind of person to endure the hardships of the job.

Through this book I will discuss varying aspects of the profession, including the different types of jobs, the good and bad aspects, the crazy things you might experience, and ways to survive the challenges.

I like to think I was an excellent nurse, but I had to find my rhythm and my approach, and find what made me happy. I wish I could say that I loved every minute. I certainly didn't. I love *being* a nurse, but there were many days I didn't like *working* as a nurse. I found my happy place in the ICU, especially once I was made a permanent charge nurse.

You too will have to find your "happy place." Don't be discouraged if your first job is not great. Be patient. Once you're in the system, you'll begin to see what you like and don't like. And with a little work, you can get pretty much any job you want.

# Chapter 3:   Nursing School & Licensing

Every successful nursing career must start at the beginning. All of the hot-shot confident expert veteran nurses you'll encounter in your career started at the same place as you, as a scared nursing student. If you are reading this, and already a nurse, then good for you. Be kind to those who are still learning. You were there once.

There are several possible entry points to nursing, each with a different time commitment and level of licensure.

### Licensed Practical/Vocational Nurse

There is the licensed practical nurse (LPN) or licensed vocational nurse (LVN). They are essentially the same thing, but just have different names based on the state. I'll use the abbreviation "LPN" going forward, but this information will cover both LPN and LVN equally. An LPN program may last one year. It's generally taught at a junior college or community college. Upon completion of the year-long program, the graduate will receive a certificate (as opposed to a "degree"). The graduate nurse may then be eligible to begin work in a medical facility, and will be required to take the LPN state licensing exam, called NCLEX, within some given period of time.

NCLEX is a computer-based multiple choice test that's administered in some officially recognized testing facility. You'll be required to empty your pockets, provide multiple forms of identification, swear that you won't cheat, and then you'll be placed at a computer where you'll take the test. Meanwhile a camera and microphone will be aimed at you to monitor for signs of cheating. It may take several hours to complete. The NCLEX is a stressful process, but the vast majority of nurses pass on the first try. If it is failed, it can be retaken, so it's not the end of the world. The successful completion of the NCLEX will officially license the nurse as an LPN.

Obviously there's a ton of paperwork and applications that go to the state Board of Nursing, background checks, drug tests, fingerprinting, etc to accompany the process, but you'll figure those details out later in school. If you have something questionable in your background, like a conviction of any level crime, or a documented addiction or mental health problem, you may wish to contact your state board of nursing first to inquire about your eligibility to obtain a license. They are pretty tight about their qualifications for licenses, so if you have any doubt, contact them before committing to school.

Being an LPN means you're actually a "real" nurse. However, it's important to know that stopping at LPN level is not advised if you really want to make a career out of your job. LPN's are very limited in where they can work, and many (or most) hospitals have stopped using them completely. Many LPN's can be found in nursing homes, doctors' offices, and home health agencies. Their "scope of practice," meaning the set of skills they are legally allowed to perform, is limited and far short of what a full registered nurse (RN) is allowed to do. They also must work under the supervision of an RN in some capacity, limiting their independence. Lastly, LPN's are quite limited in their earning potential.

In my situation, I earned around $16 an hour in a hospital as an LPN, and by the time I was an RN with my bachelor's degree (BSN), I was earning more than double that. And if you factor in overtime and additional pay differentials, I made a great deal more money as an RN than as an LPN.

Unfortunately, it's also important to know that the LPN level nurse can be looked down upon from the RN's and physicians. Whether it is true or not, they're often seen as a "lesser nurse." Rumors have circulated for many years that the states will eventually eliminate the LPN license altogether, and only have RN's. Time will tell. Ultimately, unless you want to limit your earnings and spend your career in a nursing home or doctor's office (which are perfectly respectable jobs), it's wise to continue to pursue your RN. If you seek hospital work, the RN is a must.

There may very well be ways to earn your LPN online at this point. I have no idea. There wasn't a way to do it when I attended school. We spent about 16 hours a week in the classroom and about 16 hours a week in a medical facility doing hands-on work with the real nurses and patients. There was much more time spent studying, doing homework, and doing projects outside of the classroom and clinical settings. I'm not sure how a student could sufficiently learn everything and get the appropriate clinical practice with a purely online program, but maybe it's possible. I will claim ignorance on that matter.

In my personal situation, I knew I wanted to become an RN, but entering a one-year LPN program didn't require a lot of prerequisite classes. If I'd gone straight for my RN, I would have spent a year taking classes before even applying to nursing school. Jumping right into the LPN program had me licensed a year later, and working as a nurse (although I did have to wait one semester to get in, but I took a couple of classes that would later apply toward the RN). Then I could work on continuing my education to become an RN, while gaining valuable work experience. If you have the capacity, time, and resources to go straight through an RN program, do it. But if not, becoming an LPN first is perfectly reasonable.

**Registered Nurse**

Being a registered nurse can happen one of several ways. The first way is a two-year associate's degree in

13

nursing (ADN) program at a junior or community college. This will often require prerequisite classes, which could take another couple of semesters. So the start-to-finish could be up to three years, not including any time spent waiting to get in. Many RN programs have waiting lists. This two-year program earns you an associate's degree in nursing (ADN), and makes you eligible to take the RN version of the NCLEX exam for licensing.

The second way to become an RN is to complete a four-year bachelor's degree program at a traditional university or college. This will earn the bachelor's degree in nursing (BSN) along with making you eligible to take the NCLEX.

If you're already an LPN, having completed a one-year program, you can apply for a "bridge program," which is basically one additional year of nursing school (to make two years total). This will earn the two-year ADN, followed by eligibility to take the RN NCLEX (This is what I did after getting my LPN). However, remember that you probably will still have additional classes you will need either before or during the bridge program, so it could take up to two years.

Since an LPN/LVN program is a one-year certificate in a vocational trade, all of its classes are directly focused on that specific vocation. For an associate's degree (in nursing or anything else), other basic classes are required, just as in a bachelor's degree. These might include history, math, foreign language, communications, writing, literature, etc.

Some programs allow for other healthcare professionals, such as paramedics, respiratory therapists, or surgical technicians, to complete a one-year bridge program for their RN, similar to the bridge program for LPNs. I knew a lot of RN's (especially in the emergency room) who had been paramedics first, and did a one-year bridge.

Some universities offer an accelerated or hybrid

bachelor's program, and the details vary on these. If you have a bachelor's degree in something other than nursing, you can apply your existing college credits toward a BSN, and complete 18-24 months (give or take) of nursing school. This will earn the full bachelor's of science degree in nursing, along with making you eligible to take the RN NCLEX. This is an option to weigh closely against the 2-year ADN option if you have another degree already. If you could get in quickly, this hybrid program may take the same (or even less) time than the ADN, and you get the bachelor's degree instead of the associate's degree. However, if your prior degree is not science-heavy, you may still have to take prerequisites like chemistry, microbiology, anatomy and physiology, etc. And, of course, there is always the variable of waiting lists.

I like to think the best option, in any scenario, is to apply to multiple programs, and even different types of programs. Rather than choosing one route, be open-minded to other possibilities, and see where you get accepted first. You can always turn the other ones down if you are later accepted. That is a perfectly acceptable practice.

There have been some online options that have surfaced for RN programs, although the student must still complete countless hours of clinical work. There are also online programs that will bridge from LPN to RN. I did one of these online bridge programs, after having earned my LPN through a traditional "brick and mortar" college. My online LPN to RN program worked well, as I already had extensive clinical knowledge and experience. It was self-paced, which is nice when also having to work. So, I wasn't trying to learn how to take care of a patient in a hospital, online from scratch. But it did still require clinical work. There's no getting around that part.

As far as online schools go, there has been a tremendous leap forward in allowing busy working adults to continue their education. However, in the case of a profession like nursing, there will never be a replacement for the hundreds of hours of hands-on practice that is necessary. Again, I had extensive acute-care clinical experience. But many do not. Perhaps some complete their one-year LPN program, and then work in a doctor's office as they do their online bridge program. Or perhaps they do not work at all while they continue with school. They must honestly self-assess as to whether they are gaining the clinical knowledge sufficient to allow them to practice in the acute care setting. The rigors of the clinical rotations in an online program will never be as intense as those in a traditional program.

In general, the best option is to go to a four-year college and earn the BSN and RN all at once. If that is not possible, a two-year ADN program is next best, in order to go straight to RN, and then finish the BSN later. If this won't work, then starting with your LPN, and then bridging to RN, and then finishing your BSN is a reasonable approach. It's a longer process, but it worked for me. It felt like I was continuously in school for years while also working, but it eventually got the job done. I will, however, make the claim that starting at the bottom and hitting every step on the way up made me a better-rounded nurse and professional. It is not wasted time.

Something else to consider is that if you get your LPN or RN and go to work, many employers will have tuition reimbursement programs, basically paying for part of your continuing college education, in exchange for committing to more time employed with that company. This can save a lot of money on student loans. The hospital paid for most of my BSN degree. A common period of commitment following receipt of tuition reimbursement is one year.

One final thought is considering joining the military and becoming a military nurse. I think your school might be paid for. I have no idea how this works. You would have to do your own research.

### Bachelor's Degree in Nursing (BSN)

A bachelor's degree in nursing does not add to your scope of practice as an RN. You are an RN just the same either way. The BSN focuses more on care planning, nursing theory, research, applying theory to real-life applications, and leadership.

As mentioned earlier, the best route is to go to a four-year college or university and get the RN and BSN all at once.

If that is not an option, there are other routes. Once licensed as an RN with an ADN, you can continue your education online or at a traditional college to finish the BSN. However, online is a great way to go. Once you have your RN license, the continued education toward BSN is basically all academic and, while it may require a project or community research assignment, there's generally no further clinical rotations in a hospital. It is mostly just writing papers. I finished my BSN with an online program that was self-paced.

I have not come across any bridge programs from LPN to BSN.

### Master's Degree in Nursing (MSN)

A master's in nursing can be obtained from a traditional college or online program, just like the BSN. However, unlike the BSN, it comes in a lot of different flavors. The MSN requires you to choose a specialization. Some specializations are purely academic and you will continue to have your same RN license and same scope of practice. Others will grant a higher level of licensure, and a higher scope of practice.

A master's degree focusing on nursing leadership, nursing education, or nursing informatics (among other options), will prepare the nurse for higher leadership or other specialized jobs within an organization. These would all tend to be jobs that generally do not include taking care of patients. The leadership route is pretty self-explanatory. I believe all chief nursing officers of hospitals are required to have a master's degree, at least in my state. The nursing education direction route leads to jobs as a nursing instructor in a nursing school, or into jobs in the education departments of healthcare organizations. Informatics is an evolving field dealing with the complexities of information systems, technology, and how the organization uses them. This will be discussed more later.

These programs generally do not require clinical rotations with patients. They do, however, involve projects and possibly rotations with nurses in their chosen field (working with a chief nursing officer, or nursing instructor, developing and implementing projects in a real hospital, etc). In all of these specializations, the nurse maintains the same RN license with the same scope of practice. Only their academic standing has improved.

Other master's degrees involve a step up in scope of practice. These are things like "family nurse practitioner" (FNP) or "advanced practice nurse," and "acute care nurse practitioner." There are some others in the mix that specialize in geriatrics or pediatrics too. These students have extensive clinical rotations with patients. The rotations tend to be in clinics, emergency departments, and otherwise in settings where they will work directly with a physician or another licensed nurse practitioner (similar to how nursing students work with RN's). The focus of the school and rotations are advanced patient care concepts, including medical diagnostics and writing prescriptions. These individuals will continue on to take a licensing exam and will obtain a new license to replace the RN license. I will discuss the role of the practitioner in the healthcare system more later. (Please note that some advanced practice schools now require a doctorate)

Another advanced practice route is the certified registered nurse anesthetist (CRNA). These schools are fewer in numbers, and competitive to enter. CRNA programs work differently than the rest, and are much more challenging. The scope of practice and license are far more advanced. CRNA's work with or under anesthesiologist physicians, and do a lot of the same work. They are not doctors, but they are about as close as a nurse can get. I will discuss their role more later. (Please note some, or maybe all now, CRNA programs require a doctorate)

I have seen bridge programs where a nurse can go straight from an ADN to an MSN at some schools, thereby skipping the BSN completely. These programs just take the BSN and MSN course work, combine them, and then maybe take out a little fluff from the middle to reduce the overall time to complete.

**Doctoral Degree in Nursing**

As I previously alluded, some practitioner and CRNA programs are now doctorate programs instead of master's programs. This has been an ongoing evolution in recent years. They will probably all be doctorate programs eventually. It all happens at the same schools and in the same way. However, in the end, with the amount of schooling they have done, they have earned a doctoral degree. I'm sure there is more to it. I have not done the schooling, so I confess ignorance.

Doctoral degrees in nursing can come in different varieties. A "PhD" in nursing is the more familiar version. As we all know, college professors, scientists, those with doctoral degrees in their field, but who are not medical doctors, are still commonly called "doctor." For example, your chemistry professor is "Dr. Jones, PhD." A PhD in

19

nursing usually involves a focus on nursing theory, and is an advancement upon the master's degrees that does not advance licensure, such as the leadership, education, or informatics focuses.

A "doctorate of nursing practice," or DNP, usually has training in the advanced practice fields that include higher licensure and scope of practice, such as the nurse practitioner or CRNA.

Both doctoral degrees earn the nurse the right to be called "doctor," the way a college professor is called "doctor." However, it is generally not done, so as to prevent confusion about positions, jobs, and hierarchy within a patient care setting. And I'm quite sure physicians do not like for nurses to refer to themselves as doctors in the clinical setting.
"Hi, I'm Dr. Brett Craigsly. I'll be your nurse." ???

With all of that being discussed, you will see hospital badges with all sorts of different combinations of letters after names, depending on licenses, levels of education, and other certifications.
I was "Brett Craigsly, BSN, RN, CCRN." Had I continued school, I might have been "Brett Craigsly, MSN, RN" or "Brett Craigsly, FNP."

The "CCRN" was an additional certification as "critical care registered nurse." It's a set of course work and a test that can be taken by anyone in their specific work setting. There are similar designation for Med/Surg nursing, ER nursing, OR nursing, etc.

I have never seen any program by which a nurse, at any level, can transition to a physician. I don't think such a thing exists. I used to get this question a lot from patients, asking if I wanted to "work my way up" to be a doctor, as if there was a path for that. But, technically, you can't get to physician from nurse. You would have to start right back in year one of medical school, just like everybody else. You would, obviously, have a great step up in medical knowledge, making the school a little easier perhaps. And I did work with some RN's along the way who were in medical school, while still maintaining their nursing job on the weekends.

## The Future of School and Licensing

The general trajectory for nursing education is upwards. As stated earlier, there have been rumors circulating for years about the eventual phase-out of LPN's. I don't know if this will ever really happen. However, I have witnessed first hand the systematic elimination of LPN's from hospitals. I worked in a hospital early in my career, while still an LPN, and after I finished my RN I saw the gradual extinction of the LPN's from the various units. My particular hospital also began to require RN's to complete a BSN program to have certain leadership positions. I know of other hospitals who now require a full bachelor's degree (at a minimum) and the RN license, in order to have any job in the hospital. So it is best to set your sights on the RN with BSN from the start, in order to be prepared for a long and sturdy career.

As always, it's been many years since I was in nursing school, so some things may have changed. You will have to do your own research.

Nursing school is not a whole lot of fun. Well, parts of it can be fun. And, of course, it is easy to remain motivated, as the student is excited about the career to come. But, it can be labor-intensive, with countless hours in classrooms, practice labs, and medical facilities. Often times you may have daily tests, or papers, or projects. Nursing school was a full-time job by itself. LPN school cost me far more than 40 hours a week. But, it's difficult because it should be. In order to prepare future nurses to hold patients' lives in their hands, a rigid and challenging approach must be utilized. The types of work load and schedules to complete the other various degrees and licensing will vary greatly.

Performing a skill on a real patient for the first time can be terrifying. This might include insertion of an IV, insertion of a urinary catheter, insertion of a nasogastric tube, or performing sterile care to a tracheostomy (among countless others). The skills can initially feel awkward and you may miss more IV's than you successfully place for the first months. The testing in nursing school is frequent and tough. In my LPN program, we had a routine test every single class day over drugs, dosage calculations, and medical terminology. Of course regular tests came at the end of each section or learning segment.

Then there were comprehensive tests every so often that included everything learned in nursing school up to that point. If one of these were scored less than a 80, the student was removed from the program, and would later have to restart the entire semester. And this happened. We would lose several people at each test. And, with each new semester, we picked up students who were ahead of us, but had failed a test and were now repeating the same semester again.

Although the work is difficult, it's not impossible. I know many nurses who've completed the challenge, who were, let's say, not the most well-equipped for the task. Hard work and study can overcome lack of talent or academically-challenged predisposition. It's also important to remember that perfect grades are not that meaningful. There's a nursing school joke that I like. What do you call the student who finished dead last in his/her nursing school class? ... "Nurse." It doesn't matter where you finish in your class. It only matters that you did finish. Throughout my entire career, I have never once had an employer or patient ask me about my grades. The fact that I graduated and passed the test was all they needed to know. Some nurses will have all A's through the program. Some will barely scrape by with a passing grade. But all will basically have the same opportunities in the job market. The only time I think grades probably become an issue is if you intend to apply to a more prestigious graduate or doctoral program at a larger university, or are competing to enter an advanced school, like that for the certified registered nurse anesthetist. Most of us don't do that.

Most of nursing school felt "awkward" to me, for lack of a better word. I'm right-handed, and much of school felt like I was trying to throw a ball with my left hand. The skills can be odd, uncomfortable, unpleasant, and cause a great deal of pain to the patient. You think you have it down, and then the first time you walk into a real patient's room to do something, even as simple as giving a few pills, you will stumble over your words and take too long, and want to double check everything you do. The patient may ask questions to which you don't know the answer. They may be impatient if you are fumbling around. I had patients on a couple of occasions tell me to leave as soon as I introduced myself as a student, acting like they didn't want anything to do with me. In fact, one patient in a nursing home said to me, "get out of here, I don't want 'nothin' to do with you." Take no offense. Smile and depart peacefully.

The first time you try an IV and miss, and the patient is wincing in pain, and looking at you like you're an idiot, and you catch yourself repeatedly apologizing, while continuing to fumble around... It's just uncomfortable. But, do not fear. It gets easier. I remember well these early awkward feelings and experiences. By the time I was a charge nurse in the ICU, it all came naturally to me, and everything I did was pretty smooth. I knew how to size up a patient during the initial contact, to figure out in the first 30 seconds if it's more appropriate to joke with them, or to remain solemnly proper, or brace myself for them to lash out. I became comfortable with entering a room, and no matter

23

who was there, I could discuss the matters at hand and answer questions. I had confidence in my knowledge, and was never afraid to be challenged with complicated medical scenarios. I was able to have legitimate complex medical discussions with physicians. A lot of the battle is building confidence in yourself.

You become accustomed to speaking with a patient who is healing up and about to head home, returning to normal life. You'll also become accustomed to speaking with a patient who just learned, moments before, that they have advanced pancreatic cancer and won't leave the hospital alive. You'll learn how to talk to angry, impatient, panicky, or scared family members. On occasion you may have to notify a family that the patient has died. I did this constantly in the ICU. There's no limit to the possible scenarios, but you'll find your rhythm on how to handle them. You'll not yet have this skill while in school, so if weird situations come up, don't let them discourage you.

I mentioned earlier that I worked as a certified nurse aide (CNA) while in nursing school. I wanted to touch on this subject, as I believe it's important. Some nursing schools will require the student to get the nurse aide certification before starting the program. Others will not have this type of requirement. I'll later discuss in more detail the full nature of the CNA's job. For now, as it relates to nursing school, I like to make the general recommendation to anyone who is in nursing school, or who thinks they might want to go to nursing school, to become a CNA and work that job for a while.

This certification can usually be obtained in a couple or a few weeks, or through weekend classes. Many hospitals and nursing homes offer CNA training programs, and I'm of the strong opinion that working as a CNA is one of the best things you can do for your nursing education. I'm sorry. I know you don't want to hear that. My experience was priceless, and I am glad I did it. I believe it made me a better nurse. I worked with many other CNA's who were in nursing school at the time, and many who were applying to nursing school. And as a nurse, I continued to work with CNA's who were also nursing students, and I would take extra time to provide teaching experiences to them.

To summarize, there are lots of ways to get to your goal, and you have to choose a path which works best for you. Nursing school is hard, but that's okay. Don't let failures or setbacks cause you to quit. If you mess up and have to repeat a semester, don't drop out (as I saw so many people do), just repeat the semester. You'll get out of school what you put into school. Your grades don't matter too much, but don't let this be an excuse to not try hard. Always try hard, just don't let concerns over having perfect grades be a stressor in your life. I don't care who you are. You can make it through nursing school. But you have to set a goal to make it, and let nothing divert your path.

I was in school with several people who would complain and threaten to quit every time something challenging came up. Clearly, these people didn't have much of a work ethic in the first place. It was like they were planning for failure at all times. They almost gave the impression that they were constantly looking for an excuse to quit, as if they did not want to be there in the first place. Hard work or challenging projects offended them. Don't be one of these people. Set your mind on your goal. Do the work that's put in front of you. Try to do it well. If you don't do it well, that's okay, just keep going. Don't let quitting be an option. You CAN do it if you work hard.

# Chapter 4:  Career, Basic Concepts, Pay

Some of my favorite aspects about the nursing profession, outside of the patient care part, are the dynamic and diverse opportunities, along with the job stability. I have friends who've worked their way up in a company (bank, insurance company, tech/computer company, etc) of some sort, just to eventually get laid off when the company needs to suddenly save money. Then they have trouble finding another job with equal rank and pay. They may have to start over, but the companies like to hire the fresh college graduates and pay them less, and might be less likely to hire an older experienced worker who has a higher salary expectation. I won't claim to have exact statistics on this. I have just personally seen it happen to friends and acquaintances.

On the other hand, nursing is a skill gained over time, and is not replaceable by a cheaper fresh graduate. The more experience a person has, the more valuable they become to a medical organization. A hospital can't decide it needs to save money and lay off all of the senior and veteran nurses, and then plan to replace them with cheaper fresh college graduates. Maybe it happens here or there, but losing all of the experienced nurses would destroy the expertise of the organization's workforce.

In fact, hospitals have great incentive to advance the education and experience of their nurses. They often will have generous tuition reimbursement programs, and will financially reward nurses as they gain additional degrees or certifications. There are sometimes bonuses or incentives for remaining with the same company for a period of time. They want to keep you, and your experience and expertise, for as long as they can. I received tuition reimbursement for my BSN program, and then received a bonus and a small raise upon its completion.

Many hospital systems will also pay up-front bonuses to attract experienced nurses. I've seen different hospital systems in a single city compete for nurses, as there were simply not enough to go around. They advertise with billboards, in the newspaper, on the radio, and even on television trying to attract staff, and promise thousands of dollars in bonuses and educational opportunities. I don't recommend doing it, but I have seen it done... Nurses will take a job and the sign-on bonus at a hospital. They will work the full duration of their contract (required to get the bonus). When that time is up, they will quit and go to the other hospital and do the same thing.

In the case a nurse were to get laid off, there are always more nursing jobs out there. I will later discuss many of the possible work settings, but they are numerous. The particular hospital system in which I spent most of my career had a job board that was perpetually overflowing with open nursing positions, including staff nurses, specialty nurses, and leadership nurses. There are more nursing jobs than there are nurses. That is the basic fact behind all of this. Instead of nurses competing for hospital jobs, the hospitals are competing for the nurses. A nurse may have multiple offers and be able to choose the best.

Interestingly, because of this dynamic of being able to change jobs so easily, many nurses do frequently change jobs. While job openings in a bank may only pop up when a position is vacated on occasion, the job board for a hospital is packed full of positions. In my hospital experience, we would perpetually lose and gain nurses. Sometimes the nurses would transfer to other departments, and sometimes they would go to other organizations. But there is always an influx of fresh graduates ready to work, along with transfers from other departments and new hires from other organizations. So, the job openings listed for each department basically never closed. It's sort of a given that there'll always be a nurse or two who have submitted their two-weeks notice, and there'll always be one or more new-hires in orientation.

Of course, there are less common positions in leadership or specialty areas that might require a vacancy to open. Some of these are like unit managers, or positions with only one individual, like the infection control director. Hospitals are used to the constant turnover, and so they have large new-hire orientations every couple of weeks or month, and have very mechanized training processes, classes, and certification programs to prepare new employees for work. I'll talk more later about hospital education jobs in nursing.

The nursing profession isn't going to be replaced by computers, at least not in the next generation of people. It requires assessment, judgement, decision making, and intuition, along with love, patience, compassion, and empathy. Further, it requires the physical capacity to move and manipulate people, while acknowledging countless variables that will differ for each patient. You can't program a robot to be a nurse, turn it lose in a hospital, and expect it to make difficult decisions while maintaining empathy and human concern, and while performing the physical tasks with abundant caution and grace.

You can't expect a robot to understand pain, illness, grief, loss, sadness, hope, faith, and fear, and how these all affect individual tasks performed by the nurse, minute by minute. These are not mathematical concepts that can be programmed into an algorithm. These experiences are too subjective, and exclusively reserved for humans (at least for now). Nursing is not a skill of cold calculated decision making. All judgments will have the components of context, empathy and understanding.

While some technical aspects of nursing are

mathematical, such as dosing calculations or vital sign readings, there's no underlying set of technical rules that could be taught to a computer without the human experience being an overwhelming factor for most aspects.

Two given solutions may be technically correct for two separate cases (according to a text book), however in one of the cases the technical solution is not correct because of human factors. Consider the function of Hospice. The focus shifts from cure to comfort. This seemingly simple concept is actually quite complicated, and currently could not be taught to a computer.

And, again, I think the most challenging part would be to teach a computer or robot how to do the physical tasks associated with caring for patients. How do you teach a computer to consider an infinite number of variables, while also understanding the context, emotional atmosphere, and gentle touch required? I have a hard time putting into words the complexity of physical patient manipulation. You will understand when you start working.

I can't rattle off statistics at the moment, however I know that healthcare is a growing field with no expectation to slow down. In my moderately large city, I see a new hospital pop up once every five to 10 years (creating hundreds of new jobs). Meanwhile, new clinics, home health agencies, surgical centers, cosmetic medical facilities, dialysis centers, radiology centers, etc seem to flash into existence all of the time (creating hundreds more new jobs).

Nursing seems to be immune to the ups and downs of the economy. Within reason, the economic fluctuations that widely affect businesses, mortgages, interest rates, industrial growth or retraction, outsourcing of jobs to other countries, layoffs, etc... None of them affected my paycheck nor my job security. Healthcare organizations can certainly suffer or fail and go out of business, like anything else. But, they can't survive without their nurses, so the nursing job is (usually) always safe. In a worst-case scenario, if your hospital doors close, there are plenty of jobs out there.

With the massive "baby boomer" generation now in retirement age, a substantial portion of the country's population is at a point in life where healthcare is a fixture. With advancements in medical technology, we're keeping people alive longer and longer. However, while keeping people alive longer, we're also creating the need for advanced long-term management of chronic medical problems.

For example, just a couple of generations of people ago, acute health problems killed folks. If someone had a major heart attack, they just died. Now, if someone has a major heart attack, we can often save them, perform a heart-cath procedure to open the blockage and deploy stents, and use critical care medications and machines to keep them alive long enough for their heart to (somewhat) recover. However, once recovered, the heart attack has still done extensive permanent damage to the cardiac tissue, so we now have a chronically weak heart (congestive heart failure or "CHF"). A CHF case will then require a lifetime of continued medications, treatments, and possibly medical equipment to prevent a deadly exacerbation. So in addition to saving the person's life, we've now created a patient with advanced medical needs that will place a great demand on the healthcare system for years to come, and will require the care of doctors and nurses.... indefinitely.

Think of it like driving an old car. Many people in our society will just get rid of an older car when it starts to have problems, and start over with a new one. Healthcare is more like trying to drive an old car forever. Every month something new will go wrong and will require a large mechanic bill to keep the thing running. And, the older it gets, the more frequent and complex the problems become. And, in many cases, the efforts to keep the car running will not end until the car literally falls beyond the capacity for repair (like a person dying despite all attempts at keeping them alive). Instead of the car dealerships booming with new car sales, the repair companies are booming trying to keep the world's old worn-out cars running as long as possible.

There are limitless examples of this sort of dynamic, in which we keep patients alive longer, including cancer, kidney failure, strokes, cardiac problems, digestive problems, non-healing wounds, lung diseases, liver disease, and infections, among many others. With these examples, you can see how the demand for healthcare professionals has no choice but to grow.

The nursing schools often have a waiting list for applicants to get in, and they seem to crank out huge numbers of new nurses each year. But, the job openings seem to grow faster than the supply of nurses. So, to wrap up that thought, as long as you have a clean license and a clean work history, you'll always have a job.

Of course, the first job out of school can be a little more difficult, as a fresh graduate with no experience will likely be required to enter a hospital internship program, or will have to find a position that's accepting of new nurses. There may be a little competition in getting these positions. But, it absolutely can be done, without question. I've never met a nurse who couldn't get a job out of school. It might not be their dream job at first, but everyone got a job. Once a year or two of experience is obtained, the job market swings wide open. The starting pay for new nurses is not bad, and raises can come quickly.

On the subject of a "first job," consider other factors that might put you at the front of the line. For example, perhaps you already work as a CNA in the ICU... Maybe the ICU director will put your resume at the front of the list for the next ICU internship.

As referenced earlier, an experienced nurse can generally secure a new job almost immediately when it's time for a change. I used to work full-time for a hospital, and then also worked part-time (and sometimes full-time) as a home health nurse. When I decided to get a home health job, I didn't start a job search. I looked at websites, and read reviews of companies written by nurses. I picked which company looked best to me, filled out the application, and was hired within a few days. I did this multiple times over my career. There was not really an interview, and there was nobody competing with me for an open position. I essentially just signed up to work. Of course they drug tested me, did a background check, checked my license and credentials, and verified the experience on my resume was accurate. But, I literally just walked in and signed up to work.

Me: "I saw your website and I have decided to come work at your organization. I will require $30 per hour."

Them: "Great, you're hired. When can you start?"

I used to receive frequent solicitations from companies as well, wanting me to come work for them. Once you're established, and especially if you've posted your resume online through a job search website, the jobs may come looking for you. I had constant e-mails from home health agencies, travel-nurse agencies, staffing agencies, nursing homes, and other healthcare facilities looking to recruit me. I occasionally would get phone calls from these agencies as well, and when I answered the phone, I would talk to a pushy salesman, except instead of trying to sell me a product, the pushy salesman wanted me to come work for them. It's a real ego-booster to be honest.

The following information may vary greatly from state to state based on labor laws and unions... Hospital jobs are often performed in 12-hour shifts. This means a full-time work schedule is often three 12-hour shifts per week. That leaves four days (or nights) off per week. Picking up a fourth shift puts you at 48 hours for the week, and the eight hours above 40 is now time-and-a-half overtime pay. A fifth shift is now 12 full additional hours of overtime pay, so you would have 40 hours straight time and 20 hours of time-and-a-half for the week, and you still have only worked five days in a week (adds up to pretty good money!). Or, in my case, I worked my three 12's at the hospital, and then I worked three or four 12's of home health. This had me working six or seven nights a week, which is hard (when doing 12-hour shifts), but I essentially made two complete full-time nursing paychecks each week.

Splitting work between two organizations means you make straight time at each (no overtime), but changes up the environment during the week. Spending lots of extra hours or days at a single organization will earn a lot more money through overtime pay, but it can be difficult to do the same stressful job for 60-80 hours a week. In my most extreme periods, I worked seven nights per week, and only took a day off once or twice a month. This is crazy and I don't recommend it, but it can be done temporarily if your financial need is great, or you are trying to make extra money for a vacation or large purchase, etc. I would do four shifts (48 hours) in the hospital, making 40 hours straight time plus eight hours of overtime, and then three shifts at the other job. I think in my highest paid year I made something like $135,000. Maybe that is not much money by the time you are reading this. But it certainly was for me! This required working nearly every night, so two full-time jobs plus overtime, or about 84 hours per week, but this took care of some unique financial needs my family had. I knew some others who had been nurses far longer than myself, and who made more money than me, and could break over $100,000 per year with one job plus a little overtime.

Some nurses also work in a PRN (as-needed) fashion,

in which they don't get employee benefits, and are not required to work full-time hours, but get a higher hourly wage. So, if they do work full-time hours, their paychecks are much larger than the regular full-time employees. Basically, you can work as much, or as little as you need or want to.

I worked in a larger hospital system with lots of facilities of varying sorts. I once calculated that I could change jobs, within that one company, every four months, and over 30 years never do the exact same job twice. Later I will discuss the diversity of nursing positions.

Needless to say, changing jobs frequently is frowned upon and can limit your opportunities for new jobs. But if a sudden change is absolutely necessary, it can usually be done fairly painlessly. This all also assumes that you remain in good standing on your license, are not getting fired from jobs, have a clean background check and drug screen, and have the experience a particular job requires.

So, here are the nuts and bolts of my experience. These are certainly not representative of all companies, jobs, cities, and states. Nursing salaries can vary greatly depending on geography. Job openings can vary greatly depending on the quantity of medical facilities and size of organizations. A small town with a single small hospital and maybe a couple of nursing homes won't have the same opportunities as a large city with numerous facilities and organizations. Your experience may vary, but this is how it worked for me in a moderately large city.

When I graduated from LPN school, I immediately got a job working in a nursing home. I worked eight-hour shifts, Monday through Friday, from 2:00 p.m. to 10:00 p.m. I was paid something like $18 an hour I think. I took classes at a local junior college in the mornings before going to work, as I was securing college credits needed for my RN. I certainly didn't get rich on this, but it was a reasonable salary to live on initially.

Once I had this year of experience I took a job working on a basic medical-surgical (Med/Surg) unit in a large hospital system. They were still using lots of LPN's on the inpatient units at that time. This job paid something like $16 per hour, and I worked three 12's per week. Shifts at night and shifts on the weekend each paid an additional $1.50 or so per hour. I worked mostly days at that time. A nurse will generally take care of between five and seven patients at a time on Med/Surg, and the acuity is lower.

After one year of Med/Surg, I transferred down to the emergency department, which was classified as "Level I Trauma." I'll discuss that more later. My pay remained basically the same, except for an annual raise. They still used LPN's in the ER at that time. We didn't act as primary nurses for the patients, but we would assist the RN's and perform many of the routine skills, like starting the IV's, drawing blood, running blood tests, inserting or attaching a variety of tubes and wires, performing EKG's, doing CPR in a code, etc. I spent about a year in the ER.

While working in the ER, I finished my RN. At that point, I was sort of classified as a "new graduate" again, and I had to go back through a nurse internship program. They would not recognized me as being "experienced" unfortunately. I opted to leave the ER at that point and went back up to Med/Surg. The internship required that I make a one-year commitment to work on that unit. I didn't participate in any of the additional internship training, as I had basically done the job already. I didn't even really get an orientation period. I just started working. Fresh graduates with no nursing experience will receive additional training.

I worked as a Charge Nurse on the Med/Surg unit almost immediately, as I had the previous experience (charge nurse while also being a nurse intern, ha!). I think my starting RN pay was something like $26 per hour. That was slightly higher than the normal starting rate, as they did recognize my LPN experience in the hospital on that matter. At this point I worked nights, which paid an additional $4 per hour I think for RN's, and weekend shifts paid an extra $3.50 per hour I believe. Being a charge nurse for the shift also paid an additional $1 per hour. So I was making between $30 - $34.50 per hour, depending on the particular day of the week, as a "new RN." (In case you're asking yourself the question... yes, you do get paid for all time spent in the hospital while in an internship... working on the unit, sitting in classes, doing certifications, meetings, etc.)

After this one additional year on Med/Surg, I transferred to a different hospital within the same system/company, and took a job in an intermediate care unit (IMC). This was a step up in acuity from Med/Surg, sort of a medium point between Med/Surg and intensive care. IMC nurses would care for around three to four patients at a time.

The IMC unit was connected to, and managed by the intensive care unit (ICU) and ICU director. While working in IMC, I would often be pulled into the ICU to take patients there when staffing was short. I showed interest and initiative, so I had opportunities to learn and grow. After about two years of IMC work, as my critical care skills developed, I officially transferred to full ICU status. ICU patients are obviously highest-level acuity, and so a nurse cares for only one or two patients at a time. Of course, those one or two patients are very labor-intensive and will keep you busy.

I worked for about a year as an ICU staff nurse. During that time, I worked my way up from easier ICU patients to the very challenging cases with extensive life-support mechanisms and complex medical needs. The last three years of my time in the ICU was spent as a full-time ICU charge nurse. I generally no longer took care of a patient load myself, but would manage all of the other nurses as they took care of their patients. My critical care knowledge was now advanced, and I could provide expert guidance to all of the other staff when problems arose. I would assist nurses (or take over) when emergencies came up, or when they otherwise didn't know what to do with certain situations. It was enjoyable because I didn't have to do a lot of the routine and mundane tasks associated with caring for a patient load (paperwork), and just got to bounce around to wherever the action was. I spent a lot of time managing the work flow of the unit, the movement of patients, and I was in constant contact with the physicians. At that level the physicians recognize your expertise and communicate with you a lot about a variety of topics... sometimes even asking for your thoughts or advice on a matter.

As a charge nurse I was in additional leadership meetings, served on an assortment of hospital-wide committees, worked with other departments to improve our interdepartmental teamwork, performed lots of behind-the-scenes auditing of the other nurses' documentation, participated in interviews of potential candidates applying for a job, and trained lots of new graduates or nurses who were otherwise new to the ICU. The additional time spent in meetings and training, etc. is all on-the-clock paid time of course.

Further, as the ICU charge nurse, I responded to all medical emergencies throughout the rest of the hospital. When a "rapid response" (medical emergency) or "code blue" (cardiac arrest) was called on a lower-acuity unit like Med/Surg I would leave the ICU and respond to that location. I would be the primary nurse to direct treatment of the patient, lead the code team, facilitate emergency testing or treatments, and transfer the patient to the ICU if needed. This of course is all with a physician and the Med/Surg nurses, along with respiratory therapists and other staff. It's always a team effort. But I was basically the highest-level expert nurse in the room, and was in charge of all the other nurses. And, on occasion, there would be a delay in the physician arriving, and so the ICU charge nurse completely ran the show. Protocols were in place that allowed the ICU charge nurse to actually order medications, treatments, and testing in emergency situations. In these emergency scenarios, the ICU charge nurse also worked side-by-side with the responding physician, giving thoughts, making recommendations, and ultimately making decisions at times about how to proceed with care.

This was probably my favorite part of the job... being the elite critical care hot-shot nurse to roll in and take charge of emergencies. It was certainly an ego-booster. After a while, the physicians learn who they trust, and will lean on those individuals to handle matters. The night shift physicians, as there were only a few, had worked with me for a long time, and trusted me with many decisions in their absence.

While working as an ICU charge nurse, I often would also pick up shifts in other areas. There was another smaller hospital within our system that was located in a town up the highway about 30 minutes. It had a small ER, and one small Med/Surg unit. I used to pick up additional shifts in both of those units, and the work load was usually pretty light, as it was a small low-acuity facility. Being in the same hospital system, this was all paid as time-and-a-half overtime on top of my regular hours in the ICU.

Somewhere along the way I also worked with a flu-shot operation, administering flu shots to people at a booth in a community center or something. Early in my nursing career, I continued to pick up some shifts here and there on an ambulance as an EMT, but this paid less than nursing, so I didn't do it often. It was just something different to do occasionally.

By the end of my time as an ICU charge nurse, roughly 10 years into my career, I was earning around $34 per hour base pay, plus an additional $3.50 per hour or so for weekend shifts. And, I worked nights, so that was an automatic $4 per hour I think. So, on average, I made somewhere around $38 - $41 per hour. Overtime shifts would be time-and-a-half, so those hours over 40 would pay something around $55 - $58 per hour. (The extra pay for nights and weekends do not calculate into the time-and-a-half numbers. So a base pay of $34 per hour, at time-and-a-half comes to $51 per hour. Then the night and weekend differentials of $4 and $3.50 are added to get the $55 - $58 range.

My home health work paid about $30 per hour (as an RN, much less as an LPN).

There's an army of nurses working in the United States, each with their own expertise, job description, experience, strengths, and weaknesses. There are nurses who work with a very narrow aspect of the population, such as a labor-and-delivery unit (pregnant women and newborn babies) as one example. There are nurses who work in specialty or procedural areas, where they spend their time assisting physicians in procedures, rather than managing the care of a patient in a hospital room. There are education nurses whose full-time work involves training and managing the licensing, certifications, and skills competencies of the general hospital nursing staff. These nurses never actually take care of patients, and spend their time training other nurses in the hospital. There are employee-health nurses, and their job is to manage the medical aspects of the nursing staff, such as keeping vaccines updated and managing situations in which a nurse is injured, stuck with a needle, or otherwise exposed to disease or danger on the job. Some nurses work for insurance companies or lawyers, serving as an expert in reviewing medical documentation, but never actually work with a patient.

There's a management hierarchy in nursing, i.e. unit staff nurses, unit charge nurses, unit directors and managers, hospital nursing supervisors, and chief nursing officers. And finally, some nurses teach in a nursing school full-time. The list seems endless... Hospital units, doctors' offices, surgery, emergency services, Hospice, management, teaching/training, procedural areas, home health, military, flight nursing and critical care ambulance transport, legal departments, insurance companies, law offices, telephone nursing services, nursing homes, travel nursing, staffing agency nursing, being a nurse on a cruise ship, private duty nursing... I'm sure there are many more I am not thinking of.

Nurses often work multiple jobs, as I did. They may teach full time and pick up shifts on a hospital unit to keep their skills and practice up. They may work in management and pick up shifts on the unit. They may work on a unit and pick up extra shifts on that unit, or another unit in the hospital. They may work on a unit, and do home health on the side, like I did. They may work in two totally different hospital systems at the same time. One of my fellow ICU charge nurses worked part time in the ICU at one of our competitor hospitals across town. Nurses may travel and fill temporary contracts at hospitals all over the country, basically changing jobs every three to six months based on where the agency sends them. They may do strike nursing, where they travel from outside to work in a hospital when that facility's primary staff are on strike (in places where there are nurse unions).

The nurses in more mainstream jobs may work in any number of settings. There are nurses who work in a nursing home, and manage 30 patients at a time. There are nurses who work in a low-acuity hospital setting and manage five to seven patients at a time. There are nurses who work in the critical care unit and manage the care of only a single patient.

It would seem that the opportunities in nursing will stretch as far as your imagination will go.

# Chapter 5:   Hospital Staff, Teamwork

Before getting into the descriptions of nursing jobs, I want to touch some on the support staff and related medical professionals with whom the nurse works. I initially put this chapter toward the end of the book, as if it's an after thought. But, it's actually very important. And so I bumped it up. This book is not just about being a nurse. It's also about life in a hospital. It's about the workflow, and the nurse's place within a larger team of professionals. The following professionals are those with whom I had constant interaction. It's important to know their job, what they're allowed to do, what their priorities were, and how to functionally work side by side with them.

Please note that none of the following professionals are nurses. They went to different types of school, earned different non-nursing degrees, have different licenses through different licensing authorities, and have a different scope of practice. As a licensed nurse, you will not do any of these jobs, but you will work closely with these folks.

## Certified Nursing Assistants/Aides

IF YOU WANT TO BE A NURSE, DO <u>NOT</u> SKIP THIS SECTION ON <u>CNA's</u>. Critical information to follow:

The CNA is a key factor in many healthcare settings. It is a low-paying, back-breaking, dirty, and often thankless job. I did it, so I know. However, parts of the system would break down without them. A good CNA can make your job (as the nurse) very easy, or can cause you all sorts of problems if they aren't competent in their work. A good and motivated CNA will go above and beyond to help in far more ways than can be listed here. When I was a CNA, and also a nursing student, I sought out learning opportunities and approached the job with motivation. The nurses loved working with me, because they came to trust me with their patients, and knew I was intent on learning and doing an excellent job.

A CNA certification can be obtained through some community learning or job skills programs, and is often offered through hospitals and nursing homes. When I became a CNA, I applied to a CNA position with a hospital. Once I was awarded the position, my first two weeks of work were spent getting the certification. The fist week was 8:00 a.m. to 3:00 p.m. in a classroom learning basic anatomy and physiology, learning about different medical devices and how to care for them (within the CNA scope of practice), and learning skills for performing all sorts of functions.

These include, but are not limited to transferring a patient between bed and wheelchair, turning and positioning the immobile patient in bed, bathing a patient, changing the linens on a hospital bed (with the patient in the bed still), changing a soiled brief and cleaning the patient of stool and urine, feeding a patient, performing blood sugar checks, using basic healthcare equipment, understanding the role of the nurse and how the CNA works with other healthcare professionals, taking vital signs and understanding what normal parameters are (and what parameters constitute an emergency and should be reported immediately to the nurse), and performing basic assessments of skin for signs of breakdown or developing wounds.

The second week was spent in a nursing home practicing all of these functions and skills on actual residents. The CNA's that worked at the nursing home were always happy to see us, because we basically did their job for them that day. At the end of the week there was a test, including a multiple-choice portion, and a hands-on portion with a real resident. The tester worked for the state (I believe) and administered the standardized test to qualify each student for the state certification.

Upon passing the test, I immediately was assigned to a unit in the hospital, and began my work. I initially worked on an intermediate care unit, which I think could hold around 24 patients. There would be two CNA's managing the floor. Usually we would split the floor into 12 patients each. During the shift we were responsible for ensuring that each patient received a bath, and linen change on the bed, along with taking vital signs and blood sugars every four hours. We were responsible for recording food and fluid intake, and then urine, stool, and drainage output multiple times throughout the shift. We assisted mobile patients to the bathroom or a bedside commode, and would often need to stay with them for safety. We often would have to assist the patient in wiping and cleaning up (the term "assist" is a euphemism. There is really no assisting. We are wiping the patients). If a bedside commode is used the stool and/or urine will have to be cleaned out of it.

The immobile or incontinent patient would wear a brief or use a bedpan, and we would have to clean up stool and urine with the patient in the bed. This usually resulted in having to also change an absorbent pad under the patient, or even all of the linens if stool and urine spread far enough out.

Cleaning stool and urine was a constant practice. The immobile patient would be rolled onto their side, and their perineal area would be cleaned, along with any portion of their legs and back where stool or urine reached ("Perineal Area" or "Peri Area" refers to the region on the body between the legs, around the penis or vagina, and the anus). It was not uncommon for stool and urine to spread all the way up their back and down to their feet if they were receiving diuretics, or enemas and/or laxatives in preparation for a procedure. The soiled sheets are rolled under the patient while they are on their side, and a fresh set is placed on the bed and rolled to the middle. When the patient is rolled back to their other side, the soiled sheets can be fully removed, and the clean sheets further unrolled to reach the other side of the bed. Don't worry too much about these details. You will get plenty of practice on this in nursing school. Bathing patients in a bed worked basically the same way, with the rolling from side to side, and the rolling and unrolling of linens underneath the patient.

We would assist with feeding any patient who could not feed themselves at meal times. We responded to call lights, assisted nurses when asked, and provided for whatever other needs the patients had that was within our scope of practice. I was also trained in phlebotomy and EKG's, so I drew blood on the patients in my unit for the nurses, and would hook the EKG machine to patients to take a reading of the electrical activity in their heart. Not all CNA's do these additional skills. But, these were skills I would continue to use in nursing, so it was a great learning opportunity and practice.

It's critically important to understand one thing here. And if you don't take anything else away from this book, please at least learn this part. Nurses still do all of the things CNA's do, including bed changes, cleaning up stool and urine (constantly), bathing patients, feeding patients, etc. This is sometimes referred to as "CNA work," as if the nurse doesn't have to participate. The truth is, the nurse will do this every bit as much as the CNA. Also, having a CNA available is never a guarantee. They are a major player in nursing homes, but are not so prolific in hospitals. In fact, you should see having a CNA working with you as a privilege. You will often work without them. Some hospitals do not even staff units with CNA's and the nurse does all of the work. We had one CNA in our ICU (sometimes). They are stretched thin, and stay very busy, and may not always be available to help when you need them. Be prepared to work without them.

45

If you're a nurse, and take care of patients, you will be cleaning poop and pee off of people and off of beds. You will constantly be wiping peoples' butts for them. You will constantly be exposed to the overpowering smells related to stool and urine while cleaning patients. You will constantly be cleaning vomit off of patients. You will constantly be emptying urinary catheters (pee bags) or rectal tubes/colostomy bags (poop bags), or drainage devices (blood, puss, digestive juices, etc bags). You will constantly be touching and manipulating the nude body of others, penises, vaginas, breasts, anuses, between the deep fat folds of larger patient where yeast grows, and even have your fingers inserted into anuses at times for a variety of reasons. It's not for the faint of heart or for those with a weak stomach. I'll talk in more detail later about poop, pee, and vomit. They're major parts of nursing.

I make the recommendation to anyone interested in nursing, or who is in nursing school, to get a job as a CNA, or at least get the certification, even if you never take a CNA job. If you can't handle the things CNA's do, you will not be able to handle nursing in general. Plus, working as a CNA will desensitize you to all of the previously-mentioned body functions, stool, urine, vomit, penises, vaginas, butt holes, artificial openings in the body, blood, wounds... Again, if you work as a CNA, <u>every single thing you do on the job, you will also do while working as a nurse</u>, and probably just as much. So a CNA job is like a hands-on introduction into being a nurse.

It'll also provide valuable experience in getting comfortable working with patients, learning how to talk to them, how to move them safely, how to do the various skills, and how things generally work in hospital life. Finally, it's an opportunity to learn from the nurses. If the nurses know you're pursuing a nursing career yourself, they often will explain things to you, and provide for learning opportunities.

You'll watch them perform nursing skills and procedures. You'll see how they manage their time and prioritize patient care. You'll see how they respond to emergencies and any sort of abnormal vital sign, pain, or other concern. You'll get exposure to hearing about disease processes, assessment skills, laboratory testing and results, and medications. Although you're not allowed to do anything with much of this, you can still learn a lot about it through your experiences and observations. Basically, you'll get to watch and help someone who is doing the exact job you want to do. And if you are lucky, they'll teach you a lot about how to do the job.

I can't stress enough how valuable CNA experience is if you want to be a nurse. It's hard work, and can be quite humbling, but the experience gained is priceless. I was always very happy to have put in a year as a CNA myself. I wouldn't trade that experience for anything when it came to becoming a good nurse.

CNA's can occasionally be mistreated by nurses, as if they're a lesser member of the team. I had it happen to me when I was a CNA, and I've watched lots of other nurses do it. I'm proud to say I've never done this. I have always shown respect and appreciation for my CNA's, because I was one once, and I know what their job is like. Again, I think all RN's should have the humbling experience of the CNA before they get to take on a nursing career. The hospital would be a better place if they did.

## Doctors and Advanced Practice Providers

Perhaps the most obvious of those with whom the nurse works is the Doctor. Doctors come in many shapes and sizes. Some have the letters "M.D." after their name, and some have the letters "D.O." after their name. I will not get into the differences. You can look that up on your own if you like. Upon medical school graduation, all students become "physicians." They then start their residency program, at which time they will choose a specialization. For lack of a better term, let's divide the two into "medical physician" and "surgeon." Surgeons are still technically physicians, but take on a different label.

Medical physicians may work in a general or family practice. This could be a family physician who sees and treats patients of all ages at the clinic. Or it could be a general practice or internal medicine physician who only treats adults, and who might work in a hospital. Pediatricians only take care of children, and might work in a clinic or in a hospital. Family practice physicians may do few, if any, actual procedures.

Medical physicians may have a specialization, and there are many of them. To list a few... Gastroenterologist, otolaryngologist, neurologist, cardiologist, opthamologist... These specialty services focus on a single body part or organ system. This should be pretty common knowledge. The specialties often do a lot more procedures. For example, the gastroenerologist (or GI doctor) performs the colonoscopy, the esophogogastroduodenoscopy (EGD), and the endoscopic retrograde cholangio-pancreatography (ERCP). The GI doctor does much of his/her work with scopes, looking into the digestive tract, and then using the scope apparatus to perform surgical-type procedures, like removing growths, stopping bleeding, etc. Each speciality service has its own set of procedures and processes.

The surgeon, of course, works solely in care of the surgical patient. They perform the surgeries, and care for the patients after the procedure. Again, this is common knowledge. But, once again, there are specializations among the surgeons. To list a few... Neurosurgeon, cardiothoracic surgeon, orthopedic surgeon, general surgeon...

There is some interesting crossover among the doctors. For example, in taking care of the heart, there are different doctors. The cardiologist is the "general" or "medical physician" who primarily provides cardiac care that does not include procedures. They do non-invasive testing, diagnose, and treat with medications. Then there is the interventional cardiologist. They are like the plumbers. They work in the cath lab where they use small wires and devices inserted into a large vein or artery and reach into the heart. They are perhaps most famous for their emergency care with heart attack patients, as their procedures open the blockage and place a stent.

Next is the cardiac electrophysiologist. They are like the electricians. They focus on the electrical activity of the heart, and its resulting heart rhythm problems and related procedures. They use similar procedures to the interventional cardiologist, where they also enter a large artery or vein and thread devices into the heart. But then they manipulate nerve tissue and signal pathways.

Lastly is the cardiothoracic surgeon. This surgeon does procedures that involve opening the chest to work directly on the heart or lungs. They are well-known for doing "bypass" surgeries for cardiac patients, whereby they remove a large vein from the leg and surgically attach it to the existing coronary arteries to carry blood past blockages. A cardiac patient may have one, or a few, or all of these specialties involved in their case.

The reason why all of this is important to know, is that a patient will often have multiple, if not many, different doctors on their case. For example, let's say a sick elderly person comes to the emergency department, complaining of chest pain and shortness of breath. Testing immediately shows that they are in acute-on-chronic congestive heart failure, have pneumonia from the heart failure, and have underlying exacerbated chronic kidney disease.

As they are admitted to the hospital, they will be placed under the care of an internal medicine doctor. He or she will oversee the patient's care during the entire hospitalization. The internal medicine doctor will write orders for consultations by cardiology (for the heart failure) and nephrology (the kidney doctor). If the pneumonia is really bad, they may bring in pulmonology (lung doctor). The internal medicine doctor starts antibiotics and preliminary treatments for the heart failure. He will also be the central figure managing the care as the other doctors come and go. The specialists will then see the patient and manage the one aspect related to their specialty. The nephrologist shows up, checks the patient out, does some testing, and decides that the kidneys will heal and be okay. So, he communicates with the internal medicine doctor, documents his findings, and signs off of the case. Then the pulmonologist shows up, and decides to do a pulmonoscopy. He runs a camera down into the lungs, studies everything, and decides the patient is okay for the lungs to heal. He communicates, documents, and signs off of the case.

The cardiologist shows up, and is very concerned about the heart failure situation. He begins to adjust the medications the internal medicine doctor ordered, and possibly adds some other related specialized medications, as this aspect of the case is more complicated. He decides that more help is needed to check the heart more carefully. He calls in the interventional cardiologist, who then performs a heart catheterization to take internal readings and measurements within the heart. The interventional cardiologist and general cardiologist continue to monitor the patient daily, along with the internal medicine doctor. Once the cardiac problems are resolved, they sign off of the case. The only doctor left is the internal medicine doctor, who continues to provide treatment in the hospital, and eventually discharges the patient.

Or, to really complicate things, maybe the heart cath diagnostics indicate the patient needs open-heart surgery, so the cardiothoracic surgeon is brought in, and this begins a whole new adventure through the medical, surgical, hospital, and rehabilitation process as the patient will undergo a major surgery.

So, why is all this important for you, as a nurse, to know? This all has a significant effect on the workflow in the hospital. You will see different doctors coming and going, and writing different orders. You may have questions or concerns, but need to decide which doctor to contact. There will be progress notes from each specialty, and you will want to read and understand all of them, as you, like the internal medicine doctor, are overseeing all aspects of care for the patient. You may become involved in sorting out how or when procedures are to be done, or seeking clarification between the specialties if they are writing conflicting orders.

If you have an emergency in the middle of the night, which specialist are you going to page and wake up? If you have a critical lab value reported, you have to report it to the internal medicine doctor. But should you report it to a specialist too? If so, which one (or ones)? If the patient is having chest pain after the cath procedure, do you call the cardiologist or interventional cardiologist? If there is bleeding and complications at the site on the wrist or leg where the cath procedure was done, which do you call? Or, perhaps one of the specialties is the primary provider on the case, and internal medicine is not involved. If there is an emergency, and you call internal medicine, they will know nothing about the patient. Who is in charge?

Perhaps the most embarrassing case is when your patient is complaining of constipation, and you call the cardiologist in the middle of the night for a stool softener, instead of the internal medicine doctor. The cardiologist will not be happy about that.

In many (or most) modern healthcare settings, the physicians are not the boss or supervisor of the nurse. They are coworkers of the nurse. They have a boss they answer to, just like the nurse. Eventually, the bosses of the doctors reaches up to the chief medical officer, who works side-by-side with the chief nursing officer. They both report to the chief executive officer. I have seen many cases where nursing contacted higher-level medical management to complain about a doctor, and vise-versa. The doctors outrank you, but they are not your boss. Many hospitals have even adopted the label "nurse friendly" or "nurse driven" hospital. In these cases, the facility recognizes the critical nature of keeping the nurses happy. And the nursing staff tend to have power in guiding the organization. On the other hand, some hospitals and clinics are owned by a group of doctors. The doctors are the boss there. Which place is better for the nurse? I know which one I like better. But you can choose your own answer...

That is enough about doctors. It is just important to understand how you work with them. They are generally always present in the ER. But on the inpatient units, you will not see them very often. You have to know how to manage situations autonomously, know what your resources are, know what information you need to have ready to report to the doctor, and know which doctor to call. Never call a doctor to report a patient with chest pain, and then not have vital signs, recent lab values, and assessment data ready.

Very briefly, you will also work with nurse practitioners and physician's assistants in many settings. You need to understand what their role and scope of practice is. I will not try to describe it all here. However, it is important to know what they can and can't do, who they report to, and whether they are your first line of contact. In general, they have limited prescriptive and diagnostic authority, limited capacity to perform procedures in specializations, and may often be more present to round on patients than the actual physician or surgeon. In my experience, they are often more approachable and friendly.

They represent a midpoint between the nurse and the physician. They have power to do more than the nurse and be of great value to the physician in their scope of practice. But, they are modest enough to personally relate to nurses. I loved having nurse practitioners and PA's to call.

Often during the night in my hospital, we would have one internal medicine doctor on-call in the building for all patients. There was usually a PA as well, so we could work with either. For our cardiothoracic surgeon, he had two PA's that worked under him. They assisted in the surgeries and even would do things like "close the patient" after the procedure is done. Then, we would mostly see them rounding on patients after the surgery. They were also who we would page during the night in case of problems with those patients. I rarely saw or spoke to the surgeon. Our ICU patients generally had a critical care physician on their case, in addition to the internal medicine doctor. So, we would often have to page them at home for more critical issues.

**Respiratory Therapist**

The respiratory therapist (RT) is a licensed medical professional who has generally completed two years of schooling, just like the ADN RN. However, I believe there are bachelor's degree programs for them as well. Their schooling and work specializes in the respiratory system, and aspects of the cardiac and circulatory systems. They have a different skill set that they are licensed to perform. Some of the things respiratory therapists are allowed to do, nurses are not. And many of the things nurses are allowed to do, respiratory therapists are not. And there is a lot of overlap for many skills. This is called "scope of practice," meaning the list of skills a particular license legally allows the individual to perform.

RT's manage oxygen delivery systems, mechanical

ventilators and breathing tubes, administer respiratory medications and breathing treatments, perform arterial blood draws for blood gas testing, and assist physicians with respiratory procedures and tests. They may also be trained to perform EKG's, and in the absence of a physician are able to intubate a patient (place the breathing tube in the trachea). Regular nurses are generally not allowed to intubate patients or do arterial blood draws, but may do many of the other tasks. For example, as a nurse, I managed ventilators in home health.

Respiratory therapists are a critical part of the healthcare system, and can be a nurses's best friend in many situations. They also respond to all emergencies, and have their own set of skills to perform outside of what the nurses are doing in a "rapid response" or "code blue" situation. Like the nurse, RT's are generally present on the unit at all times, continuously working with patients. We usually had one in the ICU at all times. There would be a couple more spread out through the rest of the hospital, and one or two in the ER.

To be honest, respiratory therapists are pretty cool. If I were working in a patient-care capacity, and was not a nurse, I would want to be an RT.

## Physical, Speech, Occupational Therapist

Please realize that the list of activities these folks do is vastly longer than what I have typed here. They are highly-educated and highly-skilled. I don't want you to think I am minimizing their role in the system. They require more advanced degrees, and they have gone to school for a long time.

These therapists have their sets of skills to perform, and generally may not work quite as closely with the nursing staff as a respiratory therapist. Respiratory therapists remain ever-present to assist in patient care. The other types of therapists will come around when scheduled to perform specific procedures, exercises, or testing. They are all a critical part of the healthcare team.

Physical therapists (PT's) and occupational therapists (OT's) work with patients to regain or enhance physical functions, like walking or even just moving around in bed, along with specialized self-care functions, like feeding or dressing oneself. PT's are also qualified in advanced wound care techniques, and will often assess wounds and order the specific types of wound care. In some cases, they will perform the wound care themselves, with or without the assistance of the nurse.

Speech therapists (ST's), in the hospital setting, work with a patient's ability to swallow. This seems like a small thing initially, but is actually critically important. After a stroke or disease process or neurological injury, a patient may lose the ability to swallow correctly, and this leads to increased risk for choking or aspiration (getting food or liquid in the lungs). The ST will assess swallowing abilities through a series of observations, tests, and imaging techniques, and will order what sorts of things a patient may have (normal food, finely chopped food, pureed food, thin normal liquids, thickened liquids, etc). In some cases they'll determine that a patient has lost all ability to safely swallow, and recommend to the physician that a permanent feeding tube be surgically implanted.

Following a major illness or injury that will alter a person's functionality in life, a common physician order may read, "PT, OT, ST to evaluate and treat." This simple order will turn lose these professionals to make their evaluations, write orders for care, and perform many therapeutic exercises and treatments with the patients, independent of physician involvement.

## Radiology Technician

The radiology technicians take x-rays, perform CT

scans and MRI scans, and assist physicians with procedures that require imaging studies. Radiology technicians also may be responsible for administering IV medications or contrast materials immediately before a scan so the system of arteries and veins can be visualized. Some technicians work in nuclear medicine, where they administer traces of radioactive materials into the blood stream, and then perform imaging studies with a machine that can read how the radioactive material flows through the body, and how it is absorbed or taken up by various organs. Some also specialize in things like cath-lab work, and actually assist the interventional cardiologist or interventional radiologist during procedures, much like the nurses do.

Radiology staff are highly trained and have a great deal of expertise in what they do. They're experts in the body's internal anatomy, and they're trained in how to position body parts for imaging, along with knowing the variety of angles from which an imaging study must be taken. They have enough skill to look at an x-ray, CT scan, MRI, or nuclear imaging study, and determine if the desired anatomy can be appropriately visualized. They'll often have to process the images to make them ready for a radiologist physicians to interpret. This may mean things like measuring and labeling specific structures. Radiology staff also operate dauntingly complex machinery for these imaging studies. As opposed to what you see on television, not even doctors know how to run these machines. Nurses generally can't do most of what radiology technicians do, and so they are very valuable to the team.

**Sonography**

Sonography refers to equipment that uses sound waves to visualize structures inside the body. Perhaps the most well-known example of this would be the ultrasound performed on a pregnant woman to visualize the developing baby. One of the benefits of sonography is the ability to see a real-time image of organs in motion.

This type of imaging can be done on many organs in the torso or abdomen, and is often done on arteries and veins in the extremities. A common sonography study performed in the ICU is the echocardiogram ("echo"), which looks just like a pregnancy ultrasound, but the heart is visualized, along with all of its structures (valves, chambers, wall thickness, etc). The heart can be seen pumping, the size of chambers and walls can be measured, the competency of the valves can be evaluated, and ultimately the way blood flows through and out of the heart can be quantified.

Following a heart attack, permanent or temporary damage may have been done to the heart muscle. The echo can see if all of the walls of the heart are contracting at normal strength, or if one is abnormal. It can see if each valve is working correctly, and not allowing the regurgitation of blood (backwards flow). It can see the volume of the chambers of the heart, and to what extent they contract. And finally it can see blood flowing, giving an indication of the ultimate functionality of the heart as a pump, and allowing for important measurements like "ejection fraction." Followup echos may be done later to estimate how much damage has healed and function restored, and to make judgements on the permanency of non-healing damage. This information is critical in determining medical treatment, both short-term and long-term, for patients who have developed heart failure following a heart attack.

Ultrasounds may be done on arteries and veins, imaging the flow of blood. There may be peripheral artery disease, whereby perhaps the feet and toes have limited circulation. Or there may be peripheral venous insufficiency, whereby the veins in the legs do not adequately move blood up the body towards the heart. Other major vessels can be imaged, looking for blockage, calcification, narrowing, etc.

The carotid arteries are a common sonography study, evaluating hardening or blockages that might interrupt blood flow to the brain, or where blood clots may develop to later dislodge and travel into the brain causing a stroke.

Some cardiac studies are done by a transesophageal approach, meaning a narrow ultrasound probe is inserted through the mouth and into the esophagus, where it'll be able to image the heart from the back-side angle, rather than only seeing from the perspective of the front chest area.

Sonography studies are extensively technical processes, and are almost an art form in my opinion. And, they're a lot of fun to watch. These technicians are highly trained and skilled at do what they do.

**Surgical Technicians**

Surgical technicians work in surgery and some other procedural areas. I believe they complete a two-year program to obtain their license. They are specifically trained and licensed to manage an operating room, or "OR suite." This means assisting with patient positioning, managing all equipment and tools while maintaining strict sterile technique, some aspects of prepping the patient, and I believe in some cases may even directly assist the physician in the performance of the surgery. Nurses in the surgery department will work closely with surgical technicians.

**Unit Clerk/Health Unit Coordinator/Monitor Technician**

These jobs are slowly starting to disappear, as medical systems are becoming computerized. However, the ones that remain will often act as a receptionist for the unit, working with families of patients, will process physician orders and ensure that each different department receives the correct orders, help with scheduling procedures and tests, and work with the nursing staff to coordinate the flow of patient care on the unit. With the emerging computer systems, a lot of the technical aspects of the job are now automated.

Some of these positions may also include watching the heart monitor screens, knowing how to read an EKG rhythm, documenting heart rhythms, rates, and abnormalities for each patient on the unit, and immediately communicating dangerous changes in patient cardiac status to the nurse. Working with the heart monitors may also be a single job position, without having to work with the public, physician orders, or unit coordination.

**Pharmacy**

Many people might picture pharmacists as the man or woman working behind the counter at the pharmacy in Walmart. Pharmacists and pharmacy technicians are pretty self explanatory, although they do have a slightly different role in the hospital setting. They receive and process orders for medications, stock medications on the units, prepare IV medications, manage medication changes based on the patient's blood tests, and act as the go-to medication specialist for the hospital. Nurses speak to the pharmacists constantly.

Some IV medications are stored as a powder or concentrated liquid in a specific single-dose quantity that must be diluted into a solution of saline or sterile water in order to be administered. These are often medications that have limited stability over time. So, they must be mixed and administered within a specific time frame, or the quality, effectiveness, or potency may decline. Pharmacists manage the processes of preparing IV medications as they are ordered. Doing the actual mixing of the medication into its appropriate injectable fluid may be done by the nurse in some simple cases, or by the pharmacist.

Other medications will remain stable in solution, and can be purchased by the hospital and stored indefinitely (or at least until an expirations date) in the pharmacy or inpatient unit. There are a few medications that must be administered within minutes of being prepared (like, within 10 minutes, or it will not work). The pharmacist will prepare these while communicating with the nurse, and deliver them directly to the nurse for immediate administration.

Some drugs are stored in a larger quantity of liquid or powder, and must be reconstituted into a solution in exact quantities by the pharmacist to achieve certain concentration and volume of the medication. IV medication doses and concentrations will vary for many reasons, and so a pharmacist must always be available to prepare these items in a custom fashion. Some medications are very dangerous to prepare and handle, like chemotherapies.

Basically, the pharmacist doesn't just distribute pills. Many medications in the hospital require a great deal of work to prepare, and often times this must be done immediately before administration. The pharmacy department is active 24/7, just like the nursing units and ER.

Pharmacists also work with dosing medications according to laboratory values. The physician may just generically order a medication by name without listing a dose or a schedule for administration. For example, the physician will write "Vancomycin, pharmacy to dose." The pharmacist will review the height and weight of the patient, along with specific blood test results, and while reviewing specific aspects of medical history and diagnoses, and calculate the appropriate dose of the drug, and the schedule on which it will be given (every four hours, 12 hours, 24 hours, etc). This is sort of like the therapist jobs discussed earlier. The physician doesn't have anything to do with it. They don't know what dose to use, or what treatment to perform. They just write a generic order for the therapist or the pharmacist to evaluate and write the orders according to their expertise.

The pharmacist will continue to monitor the patient each day to alter dosing amount and schedule as blood test results change. Major aspects that influence how pharmacists dose drugs are things like kidney function and presence of diabetes.

Some patients may receive total parenteral nutrition or partial parenteral nutrition (TPN or PPN). This means that nutrients and calories will be administered by IV, and little or no food or drink is consumed through the digestive tract. A disease process or injury may have caused a catastrophic alteration of the stomach or intestines, and a major surgical overhaul is required to attempt to restore functionality. Meanwhile, little or no food may be passed through the system. TPN or PPN is used to keep the person from starving to death while their digestive tract is out of commission. The pharmacy will work with the dieticians to establish the exact ratios of nutritional contents for a bag of TPN (based on patient-specific measurements and lab values), and then the TPN bag must be essentially prepared from scratch for each patient.

Another major aspect of the pharmacological world in nursing is the exact way by which IV medications should be administered. IV medications are not all created equal. Some medications must be administered through a single IV by themselves, and not mixed with any other drugs. Other medications may be mixed with other drugs through a Y-port. For example, if medication "A" and medication "B" are compatible, the two IV lines may be connected and the two medications will mix and run through a single IV into the body. If "A" and "B" are not compatible, each will require its own IV. This is why many high-acuity patients may have up to six or eight different IV's. Sometimes three or four different medications may be given through a single port.

Some medications must be administered quickly and some slowly. The physician generally does not know or order these types of specifics. The pharmacy will attach instructions to the IV bag to dictate the exact rate of administration and/or the time over which the drug should infuse. Also, it will note the duration of stability once the medication is reconstituted or mixed into an IV bag. Occasionally a drug will have a very specific instruction, such as "administer only through a central line," or "monitor for EKG rhythm changes during administration," or "do not administer at the same time as 'another drug'." A few drugs are labeled as "strong vesicant," meaning they can be extremely damaging to surrounding tissue if the IV has gone bad and the drug goes into the surrounding tissue in the arm instead of into the blood stream.

For some oral medications, the pharmacist will direct that other oral medications be given at a different time, as two medications may bind together in the stomach and each will pass through unabsorbed (among many other possibilities).

In some hospitals a pharmacist may respond to "code blue" activations, and/or trauma activations in the emergency department.

Pharmacology is crazy complicated, and requires a great deal of teamwork by the nursing staff and the pharmacy staff to ensure medications are prepared, dosed, timed, and administered correctly and safely. As with everything else in this book, do not base any of your practices on what I have said here. Follow physician and pharmacist instructions, along with your hospital policies. And, you will be exposed to all of this extensively during school and orientation in your first job, so don't worry about trying to memorize any technical details here. This is just to give you an idea as to the complex nature of working with drugs.

**Dietary**

Dieticians will assess a patient's nutritional needs and order what foods and/or supplements are appropriate. Sometimes this will be simple, like a patient is ordered to drink a nutrition or protein shake with each meal (Boost, Ensure, etc... the sort you can buy at the grocery store). Or, in the case of a patient who is unable to eat or swallow, and who has a temporary or permanent feeding tube placed, the dietician will work with the physician to order the appropriate type of tube feeding and the rate and timing of administration. These things can all vary with lab values, renal function, patient size, presence of diabetes, etc. The dietician will also communicate with speech therapy about appropriate food preparation for a patient who has swallowing problems, but is able to eat.

Even the unlicensed staff members who simply deliver meals to patient rooms are trained in aspects of healthcare-related food matters. They will identify the patient, just the same as if a nurse giving a medication, and will cross reference the physician, dietician, and speech therapist's orders to ensure the food being served is correct. Nutrition is a key component to health and recovery. The dietary staff are not just cooks in a kitchen. Nutrition is treated almost as seriously as medications in a hospital.

**Other**

I am leaving out many positions, but these are a few of the prominent staff members with whom nurses will regularly work. Healthcare is a team effort, and all of these people must work closely together to ensure excellent care and positive outcomes. As a nurse, it will be important for you to not only have good bedside manner (professional, polite, people skills) with the patients, but also be able to work closely with a wide variety of other professionals.

# Chapter 6:   Long-term care

**Nursing Home**

Working in a nursing home is viewed as undesirable by many nurses who wish to seek higher acuity patients, advancement of skills, and more action.  Others love working in a nursing home, and enjoy working with that specific patient population.  There's nothing wrong with working in a nursing home, but it's not for everybody.  In my personal experience, I was excited to leave the nursing home and get into a hospital.

My experience in a nursing home went something like this.  As said before, it was 2:00 to 10:00 p.m. Monday through Friday.  I would manage one hallway, which housed about 30 patients (or residents as we called them in a nursing home).  The residents were generally considered to be stable and low acuity.  Some were able to walk and essentially do most things for themselves.  Some were wheelchair-bound and required more help with all aspects of personal care, including bathing, feeding, toileting, moving in bed, etc.  And some could prove to be labor-intensive, having more complex healthcare needs and/or always having problems.

If anyone ever tells you that "nursing home patients are low acuity and easy to take care of," go ahead and tell them they are full of good old fashioned bull-crap.  I had some serious train wrecks under my care.  I would get new residents and immediately be asking how the hospital actually released them in this condition.  Nursing homes are often seen as, and used as "rehabilitation" facilities.  So we get medically fragile residents who had a recent trauma or stroke, and they are learning to function again (or trying to anyway).  These were often like taking care of patients in the hospital.  And you have several of them among your 30-

patient load. I had a guy who we labeled a "brittle diabetic." It was virtually impossible to control his blood sugar. I would call the doctor one day because his blood sugar was 600. The next day I would call because his blood sugar was 50. The next day it was 600 again... Many residents often have high or low blood pressure that gets outside the desired range, and so we are treating and calling the doctor. There are hundreds more examples of these sorts of nuances in their care. They are not always well and stable.

Nursing homes will generally utilize a heavy certified nurse aide (CNA) staff to do most of the hands-on work with the patients. They'll assist in bathing, dressing, changing of briefs and perineal care for the incontinent resident, transferring between beds and wheelchairs, feeding, keeping up with documentation on urinary output and bowel movements, and responding to call lights for most all needs.

The nurse is stretched pretty thin, having 30 residents. His or her job is generally to administer all medications, and perform all nursing treatments. This will include administering pills and ensuring they are taken properly, checking blood sugar levels and administering insulin for the diabetic resident, performing wound care for residents who have chronic wounds or pressure sores (bed sores), managing tube feedings for patients who require feeding through a tube in their stomach as they are unable to eat for a variety of reasons, administering breathing treatments, responding to residents' complaints of pain or other changes in health status, assessments and treatments for residents with special needs, coordinating with other therapists (physical therapy, occupational therapy, etc), documenting on the residents' needs and treatments, and working with family members to plan care and respond to concerns or needs.

This leaves very little time for helping with much else. For my hallway and patient population, I basically spent the entire eight hours continuously administering medications and performing treatments. The residents are older, have numerous chronic health problems, have countless medications, and require some labor-intensive nursing skills. This includes, but is not limited to feeding tube management, urinary catheter management, bowel disimpaction, examination of possible medical changes, wound care, immediate assessment and interventions related to falls, chest pain, and neurological changes, along with management of specialized equipment like oxygen concentrators, oxygen tanks, would-vac devices, feeding pumps, mobility devices, etc.

In the nursing home, if an emergency arises, or a resident complains of something like chest pain or stroke-like symptoms, or if the resident falls, the nurse will provide whatever immediate care is necessary and within his or her scope of practice, and basically somebody calls 911 for an ambulance to arrive and cart the resident off to the hospital. The crash cart in my nursing home was very small and limited. It didn't have advanced Cardiac life support equipment, defibrillators, or medications, the way a hospital crash cart is equipped. Nurses could perform CPR (and I did a few times), or provide oxygen or additional breathing treatments, or other as-needed medications, but that would be about it until the fire department and ambulance arrive.

I had a resident under my care who would repeatedly complain of chest pain, at least once or twice a week. Chest pain is difficult, because the only way to truly rule out a heart attack is by repeating EKG's and blood tests over a period of time, and by the judgement of the cardiologist. So when this resident complained repeatedly of chest pain, what do I do? It may be nothing, it may be a heart attack. It's probably nothing, and it was always nothing. But it might have been something, so we keep treating it like something each time. Do I call 911 once a week, and then have to call her daughter each time?

Me: "Well, we sent your mom to the ER again for chest pain... Yes, I know it's the fourth time this month... No, I can't tell her no... I have a license to protect... No, I can't determine if it is a heart attack here in the nursing home...

And, on that note, a major part of the job is working with the families of the residents. This can range from easy and pleasant to grueling and infuriating. But it is our job to care for their family member, and their presence in the healthcare process is valuable.

Nursing home residents wear regular clothes, spend time doing activities in a recreation area, and eat in a dining hall, which creates additional work for dressing and transporting, getting in and out of beds and wheelchairs, etc. This is in contrast to hospital patients who spend most or all of their time in a hospital room, in a bed or chair, and wearing a hospital gown. These chores were primarily all done by the CNA's as the nurse simply does not have time to help with most of it.

Some nursing homes may use "medication aides," or "medical technicians" in addition to nurses and CNA's. These aides or technicians have received training to perform some basic medical functions, such as vital signs, limited assessments, and medication administration. They may not have the authority to administer all medications the way a nurse does. For example, they may administer scheduled medications, but may not be allowed to give extra medications that are "as-needed" or "PRN," as these situations would necessitate a nurse to perform a more thorough assessment of the situation to determine the appropriate treatment. Obviously they can be a tremendous help to a nurse, as they will perform so much of the routine tasks in the realm of medication administration, and free the nurse to focus more on skilled treatments and responses to problems.

Being a nurse in a nursing home or long-term-care

facility is challenging, simply because of the sheer numbers of residents to care for. But, in exchange, the acuity is lower, and in any sort of emergency you just call 911 and send the resident to the hospital. A nurse in this type of facility will have the opportunity to build longer-term relationships with their residents/patients, and their families. I knew many nurses in the nursing home who had worked there for years, and loved it. They develop long-lasting relationships with the residents and their families.

I have occasionally come across acute-care nurses in the hospital who mention possibly moving to a nursing home, as it will be easier and you "just pass out pills." They may picture themselves sitting at the nurse station while the CNA's do the work, and maybe handing out some medications, and finding their experience to be easy and stress-free. This is not the case, and anybody finding their way into a nursing home with this expectation will be disappointed.

Working in a nursing home was of course the most technically easy job I've ever had, but it was every bit as laborious, if not more so, than working in a hospital. I was on my feet continuously for the entire shift, and was under constant threat of falling behind on the scheduled tasks, considering the number of residents. And, if a resident fell or had chest pain or some other problem that resulted in an ambulance being called, the whole process is set another hour behind schedule. There was not much extra time for abnormal things to happen. If a patient fell, I knew I'd be staying at least an hour late to get all the associated paperwork done, and finish all of my other tasks.

Another setting that is similar to a nursing home would be a "state school" or maybe "state hospital." At least that's what they were called in my state. I'll talk later about pediatric home health, but these may have a component that is the equivalent of a nursing home for kids who don't have the proper housing environment for home health. They may not have parents at all, or don't have a home stable enough for home health. These facilities may house adults as well, who might need more one-on-one attention and monitoring than what a nursing home can provide.

In some cases they may act as psychiatric hospitals where patients with mental health disorders are held against their will, or "committed."

I did a clinical rotation in the "state school" in my city, and it was different from anything else I had done. There were group homes on the campus, where similarly-aged residents would live. During the daytime hours, some of the residents had an individual (possibly unlicensed) care-giver who would stay with them all day. This was to ensure safety, respond to emotional or violent outbursts, and help keep up with the resident's needs. Some of these specific residents were those who were ambulatory, but also had mental disabilities and were prone to violence or other behavior issues. So, they required one-to-one care at all times to ensure their safety and the safety of those around them. This sort of care is generally not possible in a traditional nursing home. Nurses, CNA's, and respiratory therapists were also on staff to perform all tasks in alignment with their expertise.

In my clinical rotation, I followed an LPN who was assigned to a group home. I don't know how many residents it held, but it was reasonably small. I would estimate 15-20. For medications, instead of walking up and down the hall and chasing down patients all over the facility, the nurse would work from a medication room. Care-givers and CNA's would bring the residents to the window when medications were due, and the LPN would administer the drugs right there. This was one of the more relaxed nursing positions I came across. There is a small army of people taking care of the patients in every way, and so the nurse works a medication window, and then goes around to perform specific other tasks and treatments. In the case that there was an acute problem or complaint, there was an on-site clinic where the patient would be sent.

## Home Health

There are multiple different types of home health care. Some have the nurse traveling around all day to different homes to provide scheduled treatment, wound care, or feedings, etc. Another might be for a Hospice organization, and you manage the care of multiple home-bound patients, and respond to changes, needs, increase in pain, or patient death. I didn't do these. I did a more traditional style of home health, where the nurse remains at the home and bedside of a single patient for a shift. I'll talk primarily about this type of home health assignment.

Home health is a great way to supplement income with a second relatively easy job. It has its own sets of benefits and challenges, just like anything else. I spent years with one of my patients in home health, and then I had three other patients that I rotated between for about a year.

Obviously, home health involves being in someone's home for the entirety of the shift. You may find yourself in a really nice clean home, or a more modest dwelling that presents a less pleasant atmosphere. I never experienced anything too terrible, but I heard stories about nurses working in a home where the single mother was a prostitute, and men would come and go all day, among many other bizarre situations (I can't verify the validity of the story 100%, I wasn't there). I had a case in big nice two-story house, and I had a case in a trailer home out in the country, making for a longer drive and more difficult working conditions (because of the confined space).

Some families will happily turn care over to the nurse, and even leave the house for the day, or go to bed at night.

Other families will be helpful and present when needed, but not overbearing. And then some families are extremely difficult to work with, as they criticize everything the nurse does, and constantly hover as if they don't trust the nurse.

The text books teach us to never let a relationship cross over from professional to personal. That is relatively easy in the hospital. But in home health, I am not sure how it is possible if you are with the same patient for very long. I worked a lot of hours, and would often be the patient's home three or four nights per week, 12 hours at a time. It's difficult to do that and stay fully professional at all times. The family gets to know you, and learns about your family, and knows about your life in general. You spend so many hours sitting in their home that personal conversations are inevitable.

The patient with whom I worked for several years eventually died from his ever-advancing chronic health problems. Another patient died at age 13 in the same fashion, after a long decline in health. My other two patients were still going strong when I stopped working.

So, home health requires the nurse to be patient, understanding, flexible, cooperative, and socially competent. In the hospital, we're in charge of things. In the patient's home, the patient's family is essentially our boss, and things are done the way they want (as long as it doesn't violate scope of practice or put the patient in danger).

A good tip is to always begin the first shift by politely asking the family member who is present how they like to have things done. They respond well to this. Or they may look at you like you are crazy and say, "I don't know. You're the nurse." But, most often, you will find that they like to have more control over things. They know you probably know what you're doing, but by accommodating their rules, desires, and preferences, the path to a good working relationship is much smoother. I was good at this, along with being a competent hospital nurse, so I was pretty successful in home health.

I've known other nurses who tried home health, and on the first day they got into a fight with the family because the mom or dad was trying to "tell them how to do their job." Again, it's their house and their rules. The sooner you accept this, the smoother it will be. Parents and families will frequently have very specific details they want to be done their way. This may include the exact way the suction machine is positioned, how they like for the pulse-oximeter probe to sit on a finger, how they want the blanket positioned over the patient, the organization of supplies, etc. These are all things that can be done a lot of different ways, and none of them are really wrong. But we have to understand that these are parents of, often times, a profoundly disabled child, who has a high chance of early death. So, they want to control the things they can. It helps them to feel better about the whole situation if they can control the environment. Because, otherwise, they can't control the disabilities and special needs, and they know they'll probably outlive their child. The best policy is to let them show you how they want things done, and as long as it doesn't create a dangerous situation or a situation that's outside of your scope of practice, do everything the way they want it. Leave the ego at the hospital, and just be a humble, patient, understanding, nurturing, and flexible nurse while in somebody's home.

I primarily worked nights, and I did 12-hour shifts. So, the first few hours of the shift would be busy with evening treatments, medications, wound care, assessment, vitals, charting, etc. After about 10:30 or 11:00 p.m., the family would go to bed, and leave me with the patient for the night. They generally kept their cell phone on so I could call and wake them up if I needed them (as opposed to going into their bedroom or something). From 11:00 p.m. until about 5:00 a.m. things were usually pretty quiet. If the patient was not sick and not having any acute problems on top of the chronic ones, there might have been very little to be done for the majority of the night. Maybe a medication here or there, maybe a breathing treatment, maybe a brief or diaper change... And, so, the nurse is just there at the bedside to monitor for changes and address any needs that come up.

My 13 year old patient had a trach and ventilator, so he wasn't able to speak, but his mind was intact. He communicated with hand signals and pointing mostly. He was confined to a bed, and basically unable to do much anything. He could hold a crayon or marker just well enough to crudely draw pictures. Now, since his mind was intact, and he was so physically limited, this brought about a separate set of challenges. He made me play his playstation video games for hours each time I was there. His hands were physically incapable of manipulating a video game controller, so he liked to watch the nurses play video games for him. I got really good at WWE wrestling, and at a particular Star Wars game. All the while, he would be next to me, cheering me on.

We watched movies, drew pictures and colored, and he loved watching the Teenage Mutant Ninja Turtles. He also loved showing me his drawings and new toys whenever I came around. One challenge becomes sticking to medication and treatment schedules, and enforcing bedtimes. This mentally intact patient always wanted to stay up and play video games or watch movies all night, and it was always a battle to balance work with fun. He would occasionally get mad at me when I had to turn the games off and start doing routine work on his ventilator, wounds, feeding tubes, and give medications and other treatments. Plus, the guardian expected me to enforce a bedtime.

So, with a patient who is mentally intact, there's the additional demand for entertaining him or her. But I like to remember the nature of their life. Sometimes the nurses are the closest things they have to friends. They may very rarely even leave the house. They may exist in a single bedroom for most of their life. My 13-year old lived in a run-down trailer. His room wasn't fancy. His mother was no good, so he lived with another nurse who basically adopted him. But he missed his mother terribly, and she never came around.

For kids like this, their disability may have robbed them of so many experiences and pleasures we take for granted. So, dammit, entertain the kid! It's the right thing to do! Think of the power you have to make another person happy, when they really don't have much to be happy about. Never ever ever view your patient interactions as an inconvenience, or show any outward signs that you don't want to be there. For a mentally intact patient, things like this can destroy their self esteem and make them feel terrible. I can't say enough about this, and I will talk more about it later in the book. But, again, dammit, be a good friend to your patient! They deserve it!

When this young man died, I remember reflecting on all the time I spent playing video games, watching cartoons and movies, drawing and coloring, and messing with toys. I was (and am) thankful I was able to provide even a little joy in his otherwise short and tragic life.

All of my other patients were non-verbal, non-interactive, and had no purposeful movements or eye contact, etc. We played music and had cartoons on the television and things like that, but there wasn't the additional component of constant entertainment. Of course, we spoke to them a lot, and even read books, but not quite the level of activities like playing video games.

Now, back to my earlier description of the nights... Once things settled down for the night, I would often kick my shoes off, make a pot of coffee, pull out my laptop computer, and watch Netflix (very quietly) or write papers for school. In fact, I did almost all of my study and paper-writing for my

LPN to RN transition program, and my BSN program, while at the bedside of my patients in the middle of the night. Some families may be a little stricter on letting the nurse use their computer, but it was perfectly fine in all the cases I had. There was generally a chair, or a recliner or couch in the room close to the bed, and so I would get comfortable and watch movies or do school work, along with drinking coffee and eating snacks. The kid was never more than five feet away from me, and I was always positioned in a way where I could see their face and monitoring equipment. If they moved even the slightest bit, I could see it, even if looking at my computer. In some cases I was sitting in a chair that was basically touching their bed, and so I was like two feet away from them.

As far as computers and school work goes, you will need to test the waters with your home health family. They may tell you up front what their expectations are, as they have had the conversation with many nurses before you. In many cases, with electronic charting, you may end up using your own computer for that purpose. Two of my cases had a small computer that could be used for charting, but we all mostly used our own computers. In one of my cases, I don't recall ever seeing a computer in that house, and I always used my own anyway.

Like everything else, just tread delicately as you get a feel for the routine in the house. It's better to do less with computers and personal business, and perhaps let those things come later, rather than put the family in a situation where they feel the need to correct your behavior up front.

When the morning rolls around, the last two hours of the shift get busy again. There are medications due, and the first tube feeding of the day needs to be started, and treatments are scheduled. The nurse needs to wrap up documentation, wash used supplies, and make sure the patient is clean and looking sharp for the next shift.

Daytime work in home health is usually much busier. It's not "hospital busy," but there is a constant flow of activities. So, there may not be any downtime. But the stress level still remains low. There may be additional processes, like going with the family to doctor appointments, or even leaving the house for any other reason (if the patient is stable enough that the family takes them out occasionally). On one occasion I was asked to arrive several hours early for a night shift. I then went with the family to a restaurant, where there were many more family members at a large table. I sat next to the kid and just kept an eye on him through the process. I did not eat or otherwise participate. The kid was in his bulky special wheelchair, and it had all of the possible items I might need in various compartments and bags.

I absolutely loved home health nursing, and it was a life saver for me. I desperately needed the money from a second full time job. I couldn't have pulled that off with doing hospital shifts six or seven nights a week. But home health was basically stress-free, slow paced, no call lights, no doctors, no other patients who need something, and nowhere else to be. I won't say it was free money, because it did require work, but it was the easiest $30 per hour I have ever earned.

Lastly, as much as I loved being a high-level critical care nurse in the hospital, my relationships with the patients and families in home health were some of the most fulfilling aspects of my work.

I would like to include a few more thoughtful tips on finding success in the patient home. Most of this is common sense, but still worth thinking about. Do not leave a mess behind. Clean all equipment at the end of your shift so nothing is left dirty for the next. If you bring food, leave no trace of it behind (crumbs on a table or floor, etc). Do not eat food belonging to the patient's house, unless it is offered to you. Even then, I would be careful about getting into a routine of letting them feed you lunch every day.

Do not go anywhere, look in anything, access any room, open any drawer or closet, or otherwise touch anything that is not directly related to the care of your patient. Remember that there is always a possibility that you are being recorded by one of those hidden nanny-cams in a stuffed animal or something. Whether you are or not, the best practice is to always assume you are being recorded by a hidden camera, and conduct yourself accordingly.

If they put a television in the room and invite you to watch it... fine. But do not go into the living room and turn on their television.

You may ask permission to use their coffee maker. In fact, one of my homes kept a coffee maker near the patient's room for the nurses to use. Again, always clean the coffee pot and basket before you leave. Or, if you know who is coming on next, perhaps making them a fresh pot of coffee would be polite. I used to make a fresh pot of coffee each morning right before shift change when I knew the family would be getting up and the day nurse would be coming in. It was just a small gesture, but they all appreciated it.

Never ever ever ever ever fall asleep. If you work nights, and are enjoying the quiet, dark, and peaceful atmosphere of the home, it can become tempting to lay your head back and rest. One of my patients had light classical music always playing, and another had one of those nature sound machines, doing ocean waves or rainstorm sounds. You are in that comfortable recliner with your legs up. You're shoes are off. The room is dark and you are being lulled towards sleep by the soft music or ambient sound device. Trust me, it can be hard to resist the temptation to just "close your eyes for a few minutes." You think you will not go to sleep. But, you will. What would happen if the family got up in the morning, and found you asleep and you had been that way for hours, so diapers are dirty, medications are late, treatments have not been done, equipment has not been cleaned... You will not be welcomed back to that home and will likely lose your job with the agency anyway. Get up and walk around frequently. Keep your mind busy with activities or movies or school work. Drink coffee.

Fortunately, I never fell asleep during a case, even after years of working nights. But it sure was tempting many times to just lay back and "rest my eyes" for a few minutes. I fought the urge, and never let it become a problem.

Lastly, use the motto, "I will leave every situation better than how I found it." If you are washing your equipment in the kitchen, certainly do not leave water splashed on the counter or paper towels laying around. But, in addition to cleaning up after yourself, wipe up any other spots or anything you see around you. Always leave the bathrooms in the house as clean as absolutely possible. Or even just do additional cleaning in the bathroom. Having a stranger in your house using your bathrooms is bad enough. Don't make things worse by leaving the seat up or leaving water splashed on the counter, or leaving behind an empty toilet paper roll.

## Long-term acute care

There are other facilities that sort of fall at a halfway point between a hospital ICU and a nursing home. Some patients will require long-term use of a ventilator, but it can't be managed at home. Funding for pediatric home health is prolific in order to keep kids at home. Otherwise, there would need to be vast nursing homes for children. So, it's good thing for them to be at home for their development, and for the family to get to be with their child. Adult patients do not have the same access to long-term home health. That is why there are nursing homes.

A pediatric patient on a ventilator can be managed at home by a trained nurse. However, a ventilator-dependant adult can't just go home. The only place where ventilators can be used in the hospital is the ICU. So, if you have an adult patient who is going to be ventilator-dependent indefinitely, the Long-term acute care facility is the destination. Their nurses are of the caliber of ICU nurses (mostly), and can manage the complexities of ventilator care, along with other acute needs, like long-term IV therapy or IV nutrition. These things generally can't be done at home.

I had a very unfortunate case of a man in his 20's who developed pancreatitis, and it was severe enough to put him into profound septic shock, and it was all we cold do to keep him alive. He was previously normal and healthy. The medications we use to keep blood pressure up tend to also cut off blood flow to the extremities. But without them, he would have died. That is okay for a while, but if they remain on those medications very long, the tissue begins to die. This gentleman's feet and hands died and turned black. Once he survived the medical crisis, they had to amputate both legs right below the knee, one arm above the elbow, and three fingers on the other hand. So, he was left with one arm and two fingers. He had a tracheostomy by then, and was dependent on a ventilator. So, for his advanced needs, he went to a long-term acute care facility. I do not know what the long-term outcome was for him. That case still haunts me. It was extremely sad.

I discussed elsewhere the state hospital or state school where residents could live long-term, including children. These facilities have units that can accommodate ventilators and serve as long-term acute care facilities for kids who can't be at home.

**Rehabilitation Hospitals**

A rehabilitation hospital is intended for patients be treated aggressively to restore function after a disease or injury has caused loss of function. Patients may be there for days, or much longer. These may be free-standing facilities or be part of a nursing home or hospital.

# Chapter 7:    Emergency Department

Many aspiring nurses love the idea of working in an ER. They perceive that this is where the action and excitement happens, and nurses get to be heroes. This is basically true in some ways, however it's also important to understand the actual work flow. In many emergency departments the following may be accurate. For every time the nurse has a true life-threatening emergency, they may have 200 other cases that are twisted ankles, sore throats, diarrhea, or kids with a fever or the sniffles. The vast majority of the ER nurse's time is spent working with low acuity cases, many of which could be handled in a doctor's office or clinic.

The healthcare system and laws require that anyone in an emergency department must be seen and initially treated or stabilized, regardless of their ability to pay. This is a good thing for the most part. We don't have people dying in the streets or at home from treatable conditions, simply because the emergency departments turned them away. Everyone has access to emergency care. This being the case, emergency departments are often used like walk-in clinics for people who have no insurance, or those who simply can't or won't wait for a doctor appointment. Some will come in truly believing they have a life-threatening emergency, and it's not. Understandably so, people tend to visit the ER, and bring their kids to the ER, if there is any suspicion of an emergency. They would prefer to visit the ER and it not be necessary, as opposed to them waiting for a doctor's appointment while a life-threatening problem is unfolding.

There will be 30 people who come through the department with chest pain in a day. Out of those 30, maybe three of them are actually having a legitimate heart attack.

Most ER patients will be discharged back home rather than getting admitted to the hospital. The true action and heroics are here and there, but the majority of the work is quite routine (or even uninteresting).

In a higher-acuity emergency department, like the Level I Trauma Center in which I worked, there'll still be all of the walk-in-clinic style patients. However there'll be an increase in legitimate serious emergencies, as ambulance services and other hospitals will know to send the more challenging stuff to the nearest high-acuity facility.

The Level I Trauma classification basically means that the department (and hospital) can receive any sort of patient, no matter how major the emergency. This includes the major traumas, gunshots, stabbings, CPR cases, critical illnesses, burns, heart attacks, strokes, head/brain injuries, etc. Much of this has to do with other aspects of the hospital, not just those in the ER. For example, for a Level I Trauma classification, the hospital itself must have an active surgery department, and must have a neurosurgeon on call at all times to do emergency brain surgery. It must have a cath lab and interventional cardiologist on call at all times to treat heart attacks. The list goes on indefinitely. It's not just about what the ER can treat, but what the entire hospital can further handle in their ICU's, procedural areas, and operating rooms.

My emergency department had about 50 beds. Out of those 50 beds, six of the rooms were designated for trauma. These rooms were quite large. You could fit six of the regular emergency department rooms inside one trauma room. The trauma rooms are stocked with every sort of emergency supply and device known to man. These rooms are on constant stand-by, ready to receive the major emergencies. During busy times, we might put very low-acuity patients in these rooms. For example, a person with a sore throat could be treated there, but in the case of a trauma arriving, they could be easily put in a chair in the hallway until another room opened up. So, the space wasn't wasted.

Again, these are only six out of the 50 rooms, so only a small hand full of the nurses manned these rooms and (trauma) cases. Most of the others were taking the lower acuity patients, and/or medium-level emergencies, or the high-acuity non-trauma cases. When a real trauma or other emergency would come in, other nurses would come help the one primary nurse, so there was plenty of exposure for all the nurses, and plenty of hands to get the work done. I was still an LPN when I worked in the trauma center, but I was right there in the middle of the traumas and CPR cases that came in while I was on duty.

Now, don't misunderstand me on this. There were still plenty of legitimate life-threatening emergencies seen in the regular rooms too, just not the major traumas. I did CPR in a small room almost as many times as I did it in a large trauma room, especially on medical patients. In a lot of the cases where somebody cut off a finger or half of their hand, or otherwise got a limb tangled up in a piece of machinery, they would usually go to a smaller room. These are trauma cases, but are not the big "trauma activation" cases where the whole hospital is alerted and the OR is put on alert and all that.

Each RN would be responsible for four ER rooms. There would be eight rooms in a "pod." Each pod also had one LPN to assist both nurses. So, eight rooms, two RN's and one LPN for each pod. Then there was a "float nurse" or "team leader" (RN) who was assigned to two pods. They would go where the action was, or where a nurse was getting overwhelmed in one of the pods they covered. They would also sort of "lead" the activities of their two pods, and work as the liaison between their pods and the charge nurse.

There were three triage nurses, who assessed patients as they came into the ER to determine who was the most critical and needed a room and resources first. One LPN would sit at the front desk in the waiting room to receive the incoming walk-in patients and monitor for life-threatening emergencies that required immediate response. For example, I had a patient stumble in the front door confused and covered in blood. I put him in a wheelchair and took him back immediately to the triage nurses. LPN's would also monitor the patients in the waiting room for any condition changes that would warrant an upgrade in acuity and more assessment from the triage nurses. And then there was a charge nurse who managed the whole unit from a central desk. He or she would also communicate by radio with ambulances and helicopters, and by phone with other facilities.

This was a teaching hospital, so the ER was staffed with a small army of attending physicians, intern and resident physicians, and medical students. There were new nurses who were still in their internship or orientation, working alongside the numerous regular staff nurses. There were also often nursing students present. An EKG tech circulated through the department performing their job, as well as other technicians who were responsible for keeping the supplies stocked in rooms and helping transport patients. The CT scanner rooms for the hospital were attached to the ER for easy access, which I assume is probably the case in most hospitals.

I saw a lot of really crazy and nightmarish things in that ER.... People with body parts torn off from a car or motorcycle wreck, people having gotten a body part tangled up in a table saw or tractor or some other piece of machinery, people with half of their face missing for a variety of reasons (car wreck, assault, self-inflicted gunshot wound in failed suicide attempt, etc), active CPR, spontaneous abortions, internal hemorrhaging, catastrophic strokes and heart attacks, sexual assaults/rapes (women and children), physically-abused children, gunshots, stabbings, hangings, overdoses, suicide attempts, severe burns, guts hanging out, and many deaths for many reasons...

I had a lady who had fallen from an elevated position and hit her head just right on a concrete surface that it "scalped her." The top portion of her scalp and hair was cleanly cut and pulled back off of the skull.

We had a guy who had been in a fist fight with another man. Our patient had managed to pin the other guy down, and so the other guy leaned up and bit off the entire lower lip of our patient. He had his normal top lip, and then there was no bottom lip or tissue underneath. So as he sat there, you could just see all his bottom teeth. He brought the detached lip in but we were unable to salvage and reattach it.

We had a female who had been physically assaulted by her boyfriend or husband, I can't remember which. After beating her up, he inserted the barrel of a shotgun into her vagina and was threatening to shoot her... through her vagina.

We had some "de-gloving" situations. This is like where a ring on your finger gets caught in a piece of equipment, and as the equipment squeezes and pulls the ring, it basically pulls all fleshy tissue off the finger with it, like pulling a glove off. So, you just have a skeleton finger sticking out of the hand. I've seen this with entire arms too.

We had an older man who was fully intact and healthy. He had tripped and fallen, bumping his head, while at a family reunion. His family made him come to the ER to be checked out, and he fought and complained the whole time that it was not necessary and it was wasting the ER staff's time. We did a CT of his head, and it looked fine. Then, and hour later, he suddenly became unconscious and began slowly vomiting up the contents of his stomach. It was not the normal violent heaving that goes with most vomiting occurrences. This was a slow process, like someone was squeezing his stomach and slowly milking its contents up and out of his mouth. He had recently eaten a ton of barbecue at the family reunion, as was evidenced by the things we were pulling out of his mouth. It was thick and chunky, and of course smelled like barbecue, but not liquid like normal vomit. It turns out he was on an anticoagulant medication, or blood-thinner, for another condition. When he hit his head, it started a slow bleed in his brain that was initially undetectable, but later became much worse. This type of vomiting was because of increased intra-cranial pressure, or squeezing around the brain. Since he was on a blood thinner and already bleeding in his brain, having a neurosurgeon open up his head was not an option. So, unfortunately, we put him on life-support mechanisms, and I believe he was taken to the ICU to be evaluated for organ donation. But his death was definitely imminent.

We had a young girl, probably six or seven, brought in, and completely covered in bruises from head to toe. It looked like someone had beat the absolute hell out of her, over every square inch of her body. We figured out that she had developed a clotting disorder, and she was having such bad spontaneous bleeding under the skin it covered her body in bruises.

It wasn't really a medical case, but a patient did one time pull out a gun and "hold hostage" a few staff members against a wall until someone would give him more pain medication. He was shot and killed by a security guard. Of course, after he was shot, he was immediately taken into a trauma room as they tried to save his life. No hospital staff were injured. I was not present during that event.

I saw a couple of pretty bad burns, but after being intubated and stabilized they were promptly put on helicopters and flown to a hospital in another city with a burn unit.

There were miscarriages, where the little deceased fetus came out. Those were sad and hard to see.

We had the usual cases of people coming in with

objects inserted into vaginas or rectums, which they could not extract on their own. This was usually the result of a recreational sexual act, or often mental health cases. I had a patient who had a broken penis. He and his girlfriend were in the act of intimacy, and something shifted or slipped or went the wrong direction, and his penis was bent over at the middle, while he had an erection. I believe they reported that "she was on top," and so when the penis suddenly "slipped out" and was not positioned correctly, her body weight came down, bending it over in an unnatural way. Penises will bend all sorts of ways when no erection is present, but with an erection, the tissue becomes so engorged with blood it basically hardens. So, if bent while in that position, it sort of breaks the stiff and hardened tissues. This is a urological emergency and they go straight to surgery.

Psychiatric cases would come in by law-enforcement or ambulance, and the person would be screaming or violent or actively trying to harm themselves or others. We had to occasionally tackle somebody and restrain them after they attacked a staff member. Individuals who had been placed under arrest were sometimes brought in to be evaluated, or for blood to be drawn to check an alcohol level after a car wreck. They would be in handcuffs the whole time.

I occasionally saw horrible things happen to children, which was the one thing that bothered me the most. For example, a six year old boy managed to find his grandfather's gun, and subsequently shot his own hand off. Another was a five year old child who had been shot in the head in a double-murder-suicide situation, and only the kid survived.

You just never knew what was going to come through the door next. It might be 25 sore throats in a row, and then suddenly you're doing CPR or trying to stop the hemorrhaging on a patient who was bleeding to death following a trauma. I did CPR on patients as they were rolling through the parking lot on a stretcher from the helicopter pad into the ER. One time I did this parking lot CPR business twice within 15 minutes on two totally unrelated cases. Sometimes you do CPR two or three times in one shift, and other times you go the whole shift with nothing more than headaches, back aches, "I ran out of my medicine," rashes, or "it hurts when I pee." Some people were admitted to the hospital. Some people went straight to surgery. Some people discharged home. Some people died. It's just the nature of a large ER.

There were certain things I liked about the emergency department. I liked the team-nursing type of approach. I liked working with traumas and major emergencies. I liked the unpredictable nature of the work load. I liked pulling patients off of helicopters and doing CPR and saving lives. I liked the occasional action and excitement and heroics.

There were other things that I didn't like. The ER is where the whole system bottle-necks. On a Med/Surg or ICU inpatient unit, there are a limited number of beds, and when they are all occupied, you are closed for business. No more admissions are coming. In the ER, the patients and ambulances and helicopters keep coming, no matter how busy you might be. Also, when other lower-acuity hospitals in the area fill up, they start diverting all of their ambulances to our big trauma center in our big hospital. But when we filled up, we weren't able to divert to other hospitals, because we are the highest-acuity receiving hospital in the area. That means some patients with lower-acuity problems (like a twisted ankle) will sit in the waiting room for hours. One particularly busy day I saw patients who had been waiting over 12 hours for an ER bed. Some of the patients that day had already been waiting when I arrived for work. When I left 12 hours later, they were still waiting. There were times when the whole hospital and emergency department was full, and we still had over 50 patients in the waiting room.

These patients who have to wait a long time are often

not happy, and this creates some tense "customer service" moments. They see other patients, who we know are higher-acuity, like chest pains or stroke-like symptoms, go ahead of them in line, and they complain about it. But it's not first-come-first-served like a restaurant. The most serious complaints and cases go to the front of the line. And if you have a twisted ankle, you're not going to die from it, so you have to wait. I was called names and had things thrown at me when I worked the front desk. It could be an unpleasant duty station. We switched out every four hours for this job. Nobody wanted to do it for a full shift.

When the hospital would be full, with no room to admit patients, the ER would begin to hold patients while they waited for a bed to open. This meant performing all of the admission orders that would have been taken care of upstairs. It also means the ER room remains occupied indefinitely, so the waiting room backs up even more, thereby making the waiting people even angrier. There were times when literally half of the beds in the ER were indefinitely occupied by admission holds. That means the ER capacity is suddenly cut in half, leading to even longer wait times for patients.

Another problem that contributed to long waits was the teaching hospital aspect. Instead of one attending physician walking in and getting down to business, the resident physicians would first visit the patient, do the assessment and interview, and write some orders. Then the attending physician would eventually come around and do basically the same thing. So, for the purpose of resident physicians getting repetitions, the start-to-finish time for processing a patient could be a little longer than it had to be.

Emotions run high in the ER. There can be lots of screaming and crying, yelling at staff out of anger or fear or grief, and challenging of staff as to why a patient is not being seen more quickly, or as to why we couldn't save their loved one. Psychiatric cases come in and require 1:1 continuous monitoring, as they are on suicide watch. Patients and families may be uncooperative, confused, aggressive, and have unrealistic expectations about the hospital experience. All hospital life is unpredictable and crazy things can happen at any moment. But this phenomenon is extensively multiplied in the emergency department. There was some sort of drama and difficult situation every single day. And, a particularly difficult process was when a family had to be told a loved one had died following an accident. I was present when teenagers died following car wrecks, and their parents had to receive news that would shatter their lives.

We had a young man who had just gotten his driver's license, and then promptly was in a wreck. His internal bleeding caused cardiac arrest before he could get to the hospital. So, upon arrival, CPR was in progress. The physicians opened his chest in the emergency department to find the bleeding and to do direct hands-on cardiac massage. This means a doctor reached into the chest, held the heart in his hands, and squeezed it to make it pump blood. We rushed him to surgery, where they cut him open from the bottom of his neck down to his pelvis, and spread his abdomen and chest wide open. I was still with him in surgery because they needed extra hands to do blood transfusions. So I was right next to his head level and could see everything. Several surgeons were in the room and were just roughly digging through the intestines. When they found something bleeding, they would cut it off and cauterize the spot. A physician continued to pump the heart. We transfused 32 bags of blood over the course of about 30 minutes. The damage was too extensive and the bleeding could not be stopped. Eventually the surgeon stopped the process when it was clear that we were not going to be able to save him. He died immediately when we stopped pumping his heart. His parents were being held in a private waiting room, and had to be given the news.

I once did CPR on a 15-year old female while her parents watched. We couldn't save her. I was doing compressions when the physician stopped the code and announced time of death. The parents were staring at me as I was doing compressions, and had to watch me stop after the physician's directions. It was like my stopping symbolized the loss of all hope, and the sudden and unexpected death of their otherwise-healthy daughter. The mother screamed and went to the floor, and ended up in her own ER room. The father screamed as he threw himself over his daughter's body right in front of me. If I remember correctly, I think this family had lost another child a couple of years before. It's hard to see somebody in that sort of pain. It's hard to have a front row seat to so much suffering.

One important concept to remember is that work goes on. I saw nurses hide in the break room and cry, until they could compose themselves and return to their other patients. I once saw a police officer crying in our break room. He'd just come from a double murder/suicide scene, in which the two parents were dead, and a five-year old child had been shot in the head, but had miraculously survived (at least long enough to come to the ER). I believe they reported that the mother shot the father, killing him, then shot the kid, and then shot herself. This case was referenced earlier. Some nurses, like me, could hold it all in, and then deal with it after work. I went home and hugged my wife and kids lots of times, and said a little prayer of thanks that my family was safe. Others had to spend time getting themselves together before they could continue work. You get used to a lot of things, but you're still human, and you'll still be bothered by some things you see.

I saw awful things, and then had to immediately put on a smile and walk into the next room as if nothing had happened. The next patient might ask, "I heard a lot of commotion out there. Was there an emergency? Are they okay?"

I would force a smile and say, "oh, yeah, we had a little action there, but everything's okay, nothing you need to worry about." You can't tell a patient that the person in the next room just died in a horrible way.

# Chapter 8:   Medical/Surgical

The most standard of the hospital units is the Medical/Surgical unit, or Med/Surg, which is sort of a generic term for any non-critical care unit. Med/Surg units may have their own specializations, or may just take all sorts of patients. This is a common entry point for a new nurse, unless he or she gets into an internship program for an ICU or emergency department. Some nurses will spend their whole career in Med/Surg. Others see it as an entry point, where you "pay your dues" before moving on to something more specialized. It's hard work because you manage a larger patient load, and they may not be "critically ill", but they can still be very sick and labor-intensive. I spent a couple of years on Med/Surg units, and while I was working my way up to the ICU, I knew other nurses who planned to stay put. As with all nursing positions, I have full respect for the nurses in a Med/Surg unit, whether or not I liked working there.

Med/Surg patients can be any one of a vast variety of possibilities.    Pneumonia,   knee   and   hip   replacement surgeries, anemia requiring blood transfusion, gastrointestinal bleeding, low-acuity stroke, heart attacks that are several days in, chest pain being admitted for observation, abdominal or digestive tract diseases or obstructions or other problems, infected wounds, severe urinary tract infections, most sorts of abdominal   surgeries   (gallbladder,   appendix,   etc),   skin problems, stable sepsis due to any sort of infection, cancer, intractable pain, back problems, psychiatric problems, low-acuity alcohol or drug detox, amputation surgery, low-acuity diabetic   problems,   asthma,   collapsed   lung,   low-acuity trauma, long-term IV antibiotics... The list is endless.

Med/Surg is a great place to learn how to be a nurse,

and see a multitude of different types of patients, disease processes, and surgical processes. The patients will all be adult (children are in a different pediatric unit), but the age will range from 18 to the very old (of course, they're mostly very old). Some can walk, some can't. Some can basically do everything for themselves, and some are bed-bound and require total care, including positioning, bathing, perineal care, incontinent care, feeding, etc.

All patients will have IV's, and most will have IV fluids running and/or IV medications that are delivered either by slow drip or by direct injection. They'll mostly all have lab work, which is good exposure for learning the basics about hemotology, chemistry, coagulation, and microbiology blood studies, results, and how to respond to them. Many will have imaging studies, so you'll get a chance to look at x-rays and CT scans, etc. You will not interpret these, as this is performed by a radiologist physician. But you can begin to learn how to look at them and read the radiologist reports on interpretations and recommendations. Some patients may have heart monitors, so you get to learn about heart rhythms and associated abnormalities and disease processes.

Some Med/Surg units may have a single specialty in a larger hospital. One Med/Surg unit is for post-operative patients, another for cancer patients, another for trauma patients, another for neurology patients, etc. Or, they may all be mixed together in many units. As a CNA, I spent time on three different units, including an Intermediate Care Unit (higher acuity than Med/Surg), a Med/Surg unit that specialized in cancer, and a Med/Surg unit that only housed Hospice patients who were actively dying.

So, all of our patients on the cancer unit were in for cancer surgeries, radiation treatments, chemotherapy, and all of the associated complications. The hospice patients were in for managing end-of-life care, which focuses on comfort rather than cure. I will discuss more about Hospice, death, and the dying process later in the book. But, in the very specialized Med/Surg units, like the cancer unit, the nurses were highly trained in that particular aspect of care. Administering chemotherapy drugs and managing patients that have been irradiated requires additional training and maybe even certifications. So, you can still get some legitimate specialized skills while in Med/Surg. It's not all so general and generic.

You may find in a hospital environment that higher acuity nurses, like in the ICU, will be snobby towards Med/Surg nurses, as if they are somehow better. There are always all sorts of rivalries and even disputes between units. This sort of workplace drama just goes with the job. If you act professionally to all of your coworkers, then you'll be fine. I have, unfortunately, witnessed some of my fellow ICU nurses talk down to a Med/Surg nurse, making them feel stupid for calling a "rapid response" or "code blue" if it wasn't completely necessary. Again, this is an ego thing from the higher-acuity nurses, and should just be ignored if encountered.

However, this subject does still get me a little upset, having been a Med/Surg nurse, as I had it happen to me. I'll share one specific story here on the subject. I was working a night shift on Med/Surg when I was an LPN (and fairly inexperienced), and I had to call a "rapid response" on one of my patients for increasing shortness of breath. I called the hospital operator on the emergency number, and he or she announced "rapid response, room..." Then physicians, nurses, respiratory therapists, EKG techs, and a nurse from the ICU arrived quickly. This particular patient was in trouble, and had to be intubated (breathing tube placed in her trachea and hooked to a ventilator). So, I'd made the right choice on calling in the emergency crew.

The physician ordered, and the ICU nurse gave 100 mg Succinylcholine and 20 mg Etomidate. These would be the drugs to sedate and paralyze the patient in order to place the tube.  This is very common.  I, however, didn't know what those drugs were and really wasn't paying attention to the fact they were given, as I was working in the chart to answer questions and prepare for the transfer. A physician and a higher-acuity ICU nurse had taken over care at that point.  I was no longer in charge.  These medications weren't anything we would ever use in Med/Surg, and so I just simply wasn't familiar with them.   In the ICU, these medications are very common and used often.

We finished the intubation, and packaged the patient up for transfer to the ICU.  The ICU nurse, respiratory therapists, and I moved the patient in the hospital bed to an ICU room, where another ICU nurse was waiting to receive report and take over care of the patient.  Upon arrival, while we were moving the patient over to the ICU bed, the receiving nurse started listening to me give report.  After I ran through the usual stuff, he cut in and asked if anything was given for sedation or paralysis.  I wasn't sure, so I looked over at the ICU nurse who had responded to the emergency and asked him.  He stated the medications and dosages for us.  Then, the receiving ICU nurse looked back at me, and said, "Well, that would have been nice to know!"  (In a very sarcastic voice)  Then, he started questioning me as to why the patient only had one 22-gauge IV (relatively small, but very normal for Med/Surg).  It was like I'd somehow failed for not stopping the whole process and putting in additional larger IV's before the transfer. I kept my cool in the moment, but I let the other emergency-response ICU nurse have it later.

I'd worked with that emergency-response nurse many times, as he regularly filled this role for emergencies in the large hospital.  So, I was totally comfortable yelling at him about his coworker, and what a jerk he was.  He apologized to me for his coworker's behavior, and agreed with me that the guy was a jerk, and instructed me to let it roll off my back, and I hadn't done anything wrong. As an LPN, and as a Med/Surg nurse, I had never given Etomidate or Succinylcholine to a patient. These are ICU drugs. In fact, giving these drugs would've been out of my scope of practice as an LPN. I would've had to go out of my way to learn about these. There are a thousand drugs that I didn't know about at the time. And that's perfectly normal. You learn about what you use in your unit most. But, the jerk ICU nurse treated me like I was stupid anyway.

That story was one of the main reasons I was so nice to Med/Surg nurses when I responded to emergencies from the ICU. I didn't expect them to be knowledgeable in critical care, and I understood how patients were cared for there. Think about it. That's the whole reason an ICU nurse responds in the first place. If we knew how to do all those things on Med/Surg, we wouldn't need the ICU or its nurses. ICU patients will often have numerous IV's in order to receive numerous medications. But that's generally not the case in Med/Surg. So, I never scolded a Med/Surg nurse for lack of IV's, or for lack of knowledge on advanced medications or procedures.

Instead, I went out of my way to teach them these things, and when appropriate, would guide them to do the nursing interventions themselves. That's why I was very popular with the Med/Surg staff. And they never hesitated to call me if they had a concern or needed backup, and I always responded with a good attitude and tried to be as helpful as possible.

Other ICU nurses with whom I worked had a reputation for acting ugly to Med/Surg nurses, so the Med/Surg nurses were much less likely to call a "rapid response" or ask for help if one of those were on duty. This is dangerous for the patient. The nurse thinks an emergency is unfolding, but is afraid to call for help because the responding ICU nurse is a big stupid jerk. The policy should always be to work on the side of caution, and call the "rapid response" if you have any doubt about the patient's well-being. Putting a nurse in a position of fear to ask for help is not fair for the nurse, and certainly not fair for the patient.

So, one of these days, if you're a Med/Surg nurse, let the comments from the stupid ICU jerks roll of your back. Many of them have never worked Med/Surg, so they have no idea what they're talking about, or what your job is like. A lot of nurses entered an internship straight out of school, and the ICU is the only place they have ever worked. They are clueless about life in the rest of the hospital.

And, if you're an ICU nurse, you should do all you can to be of service to the lower-acuity units. Help when needed. Teach when there's an opportunity. It improves their knowledge and skill, and is best for the patient. And not only was I very popular with the Med/Surg nurses, all of the managers, directors, and hospital supervisors knew about me and my activities. Word gets around fast, whether good or bad. This sort of thing helps tremendously when you are looking for promotions. I had a fantastic and powerful reputation in the hospital, especially being the charge nurse from the ICU at night, when we are the experts on which the whole hospital leans.

I talked in an earlier chapter about the CNA experience. Higher level nurses sometimes mildly abuse the lower level nurses, and more experienced nurses will mildly abuse the new nurses (or "baby nurses" as they are sometimes called). And all nurses are capable of abusing CNA's. There's a saying that "nurses eat their young." There are some nurses out there who enjoy picking on the newer nurses, talking down to them, making them feel dumb, etc. But, this is not overwhelmingly common. The majority of nurses welcome the new "baby nurses" with open arms as part of the team, and are willing to help orient and teach. It's nothing to be afraid of. Plus, always remember that the stupid jerk hot-shot veteran ICU nurse who talks down to everybody was once a nursing student and once a scared "baby nurse," just like you. The majority of them are nice, and you can just ignore the jerks.

And one more comment on this topic of jerk higher-level nurses. I've seen multiple nurses over the years get fired for being a bully on the unit. Some of them were veteran hot-shot highly-experienced ICU nurses. I was actually surprised about one firing in particular on our cardiothoracic surgical intensive care unit. The guy was a major asshole, but a rock star in his critical care knowledge and experience. But, they did not hesitate to get rid of him when there were complaints from other nurses. Having a bully on the unit is like a cancer among the staff. It breeds fear, resentment, conflict, and damages the positive work environment. Most managers (at least the ones for whom I worked) had absolutely no patience or tolerance for a bully. It didn't matter how experienced and awesome a nurse was, their ass was gone if they cause problems with their coworkers. The hospital is a place of life and death for patients. Problems among staff that might negatively affect the care patients receive are not tolerated. And that's the way it should be.

Similar to my recommendation that all nurses become CNA's first, I also believe that Med/Surg is an appropriate place for new nurses to start. Many nurses will enter a specialty internship out of school (ER, ICU, Operating Room, etc), but I feel like they miss part of the learning experience to not start at the "bottom" on the acuity level and work their way up as I did. Being a CNA made me a better nurse. Being a nursing home nurse made me a better Med/Surg nurse. Being an LPN made me a better RN. Being a Med/Surg Nurse made me a better emergency room and ICU nurse.

I apologize for spending so much time on something negative, like bullying. But I intended to write about the nursing experience, and not just the technical aspects of the profession. This is something you'll come across in a hospital. But, again, don't let the jerks get to you. Most people will be very pleasant to work with.

Overall, Med/Surg is a great place to work for many nurses, and it really makes up the biggest majority of staff nurse positions in a hospital. Med/Surg nurses vastly outnumber ICU nurses. Some will say that they enjoy working in Med/Surg because most of their patients are awake and they can have a working relationship. They don't like that so many of the patients in ICU are sedated or comatose and on ventilators and other life-support apparatus. Some nurses are just not comfortable taking on the higher-acuity stuff in the ICU. I met several Med/Surg nurses who had been doing it for 15 years or more. As stated earlier, every nurse will have his or her own preference, and will like different units. Working one unit versus another unit doesn't mean that somebody is smarter or more capable. I believe most any nurse can be trained to work as a Med/Surg nurse or an ICU nurse, so avoid social dynamics where your peers act otherwise. All nursing units are different, but equal.

**A day in the life of a Med/Surg nurse**

My Med/Surg experience will clearly not represent all Med/Surg units. There is a great deal of variety among patient loads and acuity levels from one hospital to another. My particular Med/Surg unit was pretty high acuity. When I moved to a different hospital within the system to work in the IMC and ICU, I found that their Med/Surg units were much lower acuity. They were sending patients to the ICU who were no sicker that the patients on my previous Med/Surg unit.

When I worked days in Med/Surg, life was pretty

crazy. The overlap for report and handoff would be from 0645 to 0715 between the night and oncoming day nurses. I generally found that once report was over at 0715, I hit the floor running. I would need to check in on each of my five, six, or seven patients, make sure nobody had a serious problem that required immediate attention, and then begin working my way through the morning vital signs, assessments, medications, treatments, etc for each patient. Meanwhile the patients received their breakfast, and there was often something more to be done. Some patients required assistance cutting up food, some required a staff member to feed them, some needed supplements prepared with their meal, and some just wanted to complain about the food. We had two CNA's on this 38-bed unit. So, they couldn't do all of the feeding. Nurses had to do a lot of the meal-related tasks too.

As the morning was starting, the army of physicians and residents/interns/medical students began to round on the patients, and would write new orders, change orders, or write orders to discharge or transfer. With each new order set, there would be changes to patient medications, treatments, testing, procedures, and/or meals. Many times orders might have to be clarified with the physician if they were not written clearly, or if the nurse had reason to question the appropriateness of the order. For example, "are you sure you want to give this med to a patient whose kidney's don't work?" By then the physician was gone and had to be paged.

So, as fast as I could get vitals, perform head-to-toe assessments, start administering medications and performing treatments, assisting with meals, assisting with trips to the toilet, assisting with brief changes for incontinent patients, along with answering call lights and responding to every need, the physician would roll in and change everything up. Just when I began to almost catch up, one or two patients would need to discharge. This was a whole process to remove IV's and get them dressed, coordinate with a wheelchair van or ambulance or their family to provide transportation, call report to a receiving facility (like back to the nursing home) if applicable, provide teaching on the discharge instructions, get the paperwork all signed, and then physically get them out of the unit and into a wheelchair van or ambulance or car. Then more work had to be done in the chart to close out care plans and document the discharge process (along with all of the other shift assessment documentation and other chores).

Once the patient was out of the room, housekeeping would show up and have the room clean 20 minutes later. As soon as the room was clean, the emergency department was calling report and wanted to send up the next admission. Meanwhile, lunch was being served, with all of the work assisting patients with the meal. Medications and treatments were due, orders continued to change, patients continued to have pain or other problems and needed PRN medications (as-needed, like pain medicine), patients continued to push the call light for any one of a thousand possible needs, briefs needed to be changed on the incontinent patient, the immobile patients had to be repositioned in bed and have a brief change at least every two hours, coworkers wanted to go to lunch and were asking for someone to watch their patients, patients were coming and going for testing and procedures, families and/or patients had questions/concerns/complaints, and there had not even been time to start the charting and nursing documentation yet.

When the new patient arrived, and we were still doing all of these other tasks with the other patients, the new patient would require a mountain of paperwork to be completed, assessments, vital signs, an entire new set of orders, questions/concerns/complaints, families calling to check on them, starting IV drip medications, and applying all of the compression stockings and/or pneumatic compression devices and/or a heart monitor and/or other special equipment.

Meanwhile, another patient was ready for discharge, and the other four or five patients would continue to have their orders, medications, treatments, tests, procedures, and problems as the afternoon continued.

Upon finally getting the admission settled, and getting the next discharge out of the hospital, the discharged room was cleaned and the next admission was on the way. Supper arrived, and the process began with early-evening medications, treatments, tests, procedures, problems, questions, pain, repositioning, brief changes, and assistance with the meal. The new admission arrived, and so that lengthy process started again. As they were finally settled and all of their tasks and orders were caught up, the last hour or so of the shift was spent trying to catch up any remaining tasks that were behind.

When shift change arrived at 1900 (7:00 pm), report and care was handed off, and the day nurses were relieved of duty. But, on a really busy day, we likely hadn't even touched our general charting and documentation for all of the patients, and possibly the admissions, and possibly even the discharges. So, we sat at a computer and spent the next hour charting (after our shift was over).

Some days are busier than others. Some days will feel like you run so fast and stay so busy, that you have trouble finding three minutes to go to the bathroom. I wore a pedometer one time on the unit to measure the distance I walked... six miles. Six miles up and down a few short hallways and between adjacent rooms, over 12 hours. Sometimes it can be difficult to squeeze in a lunch break.

Other days aren't so busy, and maybe the unit isn't even full. Discharges are not immediately replaced by admissions, as the ER is empty. And a nurse may even have one or two open rooms for the whole shift, never actually having a full load of patients. The nurse may have a surprising amount of free time. Staffing may vary, and if the unit is short a nurse, then everybody has to take an extra patient. If the unit is fully staffed, and there are enough empty rooms, then a nurse may get sent home and either be cancelled for the day or will be on-call in case admissions arrive. Or, extra nurses may be "floated" to another department where staffing is short. This is a very common practice, and is widely despised by all nurses. It sucks to have to go and work on a strange unit.

I used to pick up shifts in a small hospital located in the next small town up the highway, but it was still in the same hospital system. They had one Med/Surg unit, which I found to be particularly easy and stress-free. I worked there some in both the ER and Med/Surg units while I was an ICU charge nurse at my hospital. It was just a small and slow-paced facility. Many of the patients there were of particularly low acuity, simply because the overall acuity of the hospital was low. There was no IMC or ICU, and the ER staff was generally four or five nurses during the day and down to two nurses at night.

So, if you find yourself in the world of Med/Surg, you could be on a crazy-busy unit like my early experiences, or you could be on a really relaxed low-acuity unit. Or, I suppose, anywhere in between. But always remember, if you find yourself in an environment that is intense and challenging, even if you don't enjoy it, appreciate the experience. It will make you a better nurse.

I will discuss life in the ICU in a later chapter, and compare it with this explanation of life in Med/Surg. But, Med/Surg often requires a lot of work, much of which may not be terribly advanced. However, much of it may feel like you're just running room to room non-stop, and struggling to keep up with scheduled medications, treatments, charting, etc. The patients are less advanced, and the nursing expertise is lower, but the workload is heavily stretched between lots of patients. The ICU is sort of the opposite. The nurse may have only one or two patients, but they'll work tirelessly doing highly advanced nursing activities. They may not be running room to room continuously, but they're constantly working on their one or two patients. I always found this to be less stressful for me. I could work hard, but all of my attention was focused on one or two rooms only. There was never that realization that you've been so busy you haven't seen one of your six or seven patients in hours. There's not the continuous running from room to room to answer call lights. Instead, you are constantly challenged in your knowledge, skill, and decision-making, rather than being challenged by stretching yourself so thin between so many patients.

I don't want to come across as being negative about my busy experiences in Med/Surg. Some nurses love the fast-paced environment. And it's not ever intolerably busy. The work always gets done. And, again, it's a great place to really learn how to be a nurse, how to manage your time, how to manage a larger patient load, and to gain so much of the basic and intermediate-level nursing knowledge and experience.

# Chapter 9:   Intermediate & Critical Care

As discussed, my goal was always to get into critical care, and I eventually did.  So, I am partial to this area, but remember that no one unit is better than another.

**Intensive Care Unit**
An ICU can vary greatly depending on the size of the hospital, along with the particular hospital's capabilities.  For example, a smaller hospital may have a single ICU that takes on most all critical care cases that the hospital handles.  This might include medical patients (infections, diabetic problems, sepsis, renal problems, liver problems, etc).  It may also include some trauma, neurology, and cardiology, if the hospital takes those kinds of patients.  When I worked in the Level I Trauma Center in a large hospital, there were several different ICU's...    medical, surgical/trauma, neurology, cardio-thoracic, pediatric, neonatal...

Medical patients, like the ones listed above, go to the Medical ICU.  Strokes, brain injuries, and other neurological problems go to neuro ICU.  Patients who have had heart attacks and are unstable, or who have had open chest surgeries on their heart or lungs, or who are dependant on an external device to circulate their blood for them, will go to cardiothoracic ICU.  Severe trauma and critical surgical patients go to the surgical/trauma ICU.  And of course kids go to the Pediatric ICU, and newborns go to the Neonatal ICU.

Some of the lower-acuity ICU patients (still very sick but becoming more stable) will be awake and can talk and do things for themselves and are fairly easy to care for.  These typically will be downgraded to Med/Surg at the point they are this stable.

On the other extreme are patients who have all of, or some combination of the following: a machine breathing for them, a machine circulating their blood for them, a machine pulling out blood and filtering it and then returning it to the body (dialysis) since their kidneys are shut down, an assortment of pleural and mediastinal chest tubes to drain air and fluid and blood from around the lungs and heart, urinary catheter, pulmonary artery catheter inserted into the jugular vein of the neck and threaded through the heart and into the arteries of the lungs, an arterial line in their groin or wrist, numerous IV's, nasogastric or orogastric tube that runs down their esophagus into the stomach providing feeding or evacuating the stomach if needed, a central line threaded into the vena cava (major central vein in the abdomen and chest), possibly a surgically opened abdomen or chest (yes, still opened up wide, and covered with a sheet of sterile plastic), rectal tube, device to manually warm or cool the body, external pacemakers that have wires threaded through a hole in the chest and attached directly to the heart, and anywhere from five to 10 to 15 different continuous IV medications running (sedation, pain control, chemical paralysis, antibiotics, insulin, dextrose, medications to open the arteries up or clamp them down, blood products, medications to control heart rate/rhythm and/or increase or decrease the pumping of the heart, medications to slow or speed blood clotting...) The list goes way beyond these few medications and devices.

The nurse will be continuously monitoring and calculating advanced hemodynamic readings, as they are taken from the various catheters inserted into the arteries, veins, heart, lungs, along with the heart monitor, and vital signs, and body temperature, and all of the possible physical assessment data.... (Again, the list goes way beyond these few items).

The nurse must be able to accurately measure the

various components of advanced hemodynamics, be able to operate all of the equipment correctly, and be able to autonomously make changes to everything continuously based on vitals, hemodynamic readings, blood tests, imaging studies, etc. And each time an adjustment is made to a machine or a medication, it will correct one problem while simultaneously changing some other parameter. For example, a hypothetical patient needs his coronary arteries dilated following a heart attack, so an infusion of IV nitroglycerin is started, but this lowers blood pressure, so vasopressin and/or levophed and/or ephinephrine and/or neosynephrine are started or increased to constrict the peripheral arteries and increase blood pressure, or albumin is infused to shift fluid from extra-vascular to intra-vascular spaces to increase circulating volume, and the increase in blood pressure decreases cardiac output in the weakened heart by increasing peripheral artery resistance, so dobutamine is started or increased to make the heart pump harder, but the dobutamine causes electrical irritability so the heart rhythm changes, so amiodarone is started or increased to calm the heart down. Then, the IV insulin that is running shifts too much potassium from the extracellular to the intracellular spaces, so potassium replacement is necessary and requires continuous frequent blood test to check levels and adjust replacement dosing. Potassium is just one example. There are lots of electrolytes to be monitored and replaced.

Then pulmonary artery pressure is noted to have increased due to all of the other medications to increase heart rate and cardiac output, so nitric oxide is connected into the flow of the ventilator to dilate these arteries. The blood pressure begins to decrease, so an arterial blood gas is run and it shows that the patient's blood pH has become too acidic and their carbon dioxide level is too high, so the rate on the ventilator is turned up to blow off more carbon dioxide, thereby reducing carbonic acid in the body, and correcting the pH. Also an infusion of sodium bicarbonate may be started or increased to counteract the acidosis that is occurring. Once the pH is corrected, the blood pressure responds more appropriately to the other medications.

Then, for no good reason, just because cardiac patients have an angry heart, the rhythm changes to ventricular tachycardia, and blood flow is lost. So, the nurse delivers a shock from the defibrillator (like you see on TV.... "Clear!" Wham!). If the patient had heart surgery for the heart attack he or she will already have blood clotting problems and potential anemia. This just happens with that surgery. Blood tests for a variety of perspectives of the blood clotting cascade will be done frequently, and the nurse will transfuse blood, or platelets, or plasma, or albumin. Medication may be running to slow clotting of the blood (a blood thinner as it is often called), and so frequent blood tests are performed in order to adjust dosing... (As said before, the list goes way beyond these few items)

I am just rambling on now, so forgive the lengthy example, and forgive me for explaining it all in such a disjointed and grammatically-incorrect way. But this gives the experiential aroma of what ICU nurses do. There are seemingly limitless possible problems and combinations of problems, along with treatments and medications. The above lists and situations are only a short part of the longer list of things we do. Further, and please pay attention because this is important, the nurses and respiratory therapists often do all of this without the presence of a physician. We have orders that give general parameters and give us the tools we can use. But the nurse makes all the decisions and freely uses those tools.

I worked nights in an ICU where we took patients who had open heart surgery. They are far too unstable to go to the post-op area. They come straight to the ICU from the operating table. They will be deeply sedated, they will be on a ventilator, they will have some combination of 10 or 15 different IV medications running, they will have chest tubes and external pacemakers and may have intra-aortic balloon pump or impella, may be on continuous dialysis, or any number of other processes. We would get these patients at shift change from the OR, just as we were starting our night shift. The surgeon would come by and check on the patient in the room. He would then write pages of orders for every different medication, treatment, blood transfusion, and test we might need. Then he goes home and goes to bed.

The nurse takes over from there, and just knows how to do everything. There are written protocols for some of the responses and changes, but many are just done by the nurse's best judgement, estimation, and intuition. If you have titrated levophed for blood pressure support enough times, you get a feel for how patients respond, and in what period of time.

This also brings up another point. You don't just blindly give the medications because the doctor said so. You know what each one does, you know exactly what receptors it hits in the body, you know the half life, you know the time to peak effect, you know the expected side effects, you know how it will react with or affect other medications, and you know exactly what hemodynamic parameters to watch. You know how to stand there for 12 hours and continuously assess the patient, assess the hemodynamics, manipulate medications, run blood tests and know how to interpret and respond to the results. A single nurse can spend 12 straight hours of continuous work like this on one patient, without having downtime or being able to put things on cruise control, and mostly relying on their own knowledge, judgement, experience, study, practice, expertise, and intuition to keep the patient alive.

I have heard non-medical people make the assumption that nurses just follow orders, as if they do not think for themselves. In reality, in Med/Surg, and especially in the ICU, there are no doctors standing around telling you what to do. You have autonomy as the nurse, and you make life and death decisions for the patient. You are not just the doctor's helper. You are a highly trained and highly skilled medical professional with advanced medical knowledge. Do not ever let someone tell you otherwise. The above hypothetical example should prove that point.

Nurses in the ICU will generally have one to three patients, depending on acuity. With a fresh open-heart surgery patient, a patient being made artificially hypothermic after CPR, a patient on continuous dialysis, or a patient with a intra-aortic balloon pump (among many other possible scenarios), the nurse will only have this one patient to care for. They will spend 12 hours in that patient's room, or at the computer station directly outside of the room (where the patient can be seen through a window, and where the heart monitor display shows on a screen outside the room). If they need to make a bathroom trip or take a lunch break, they will ask a less-busy nurse or the charge nurse to come stay with their patient for a few minutes. The patient is never left alone. Too many things can go wrong, and it can happen fast. A nurse must be on the ready at all times to respond to changes.

For other less-complex patients, the nurse may have two at a time, or even three if staffing is short or the patients are really easy to care for.

I am not going to spend too much time trying to tell specific stories about ICU patients. The complex example I gave earlier is a pretty good representation of an ICU patient. The dynamic is different from the ER. The ER is more unpredictable and is all about stabilizing patients to pass them on to the inpatient units or procedural areas. The crazy stories, like those I discussed in the ER chapter of this book, tend to be far more dramatic in that setting. The same patients eventually end up in the ICU, but by that time they are on all of the life-support machines and the strategic calculated "chess match" begins to keep them alive for the coming hours and days. But, just like the ER, I did CPR constantly in the ICU. We had plenty of emergencies there.

## Intermediate Care Unit or Progressive Care Unit

Intermediate or progressive care is basically the halfway point between Med/Surg and ICU. The patients are too sick and/or complicated for Med/Surg, but just don't quite have enough problems to make full ICU status. This may also be where patients in the ICU will be relocated when they have become stable enough to be downgraded, but require closer monitoring than what can be done on Med/Surg.

The skill level of the nurses is also at an intermediate point. They do more than Med/Surg nurses, but less than ICU nurses in the way of complex patients and more advanced medications, procedures, and equipment.

For me, intermediate care was my stepping stone to move from Med/Surg to ICU. These nurses will usually have three or four patients.

# Chapter 10:   Specialty Areas

There are several specialized inpatient units in a hospital, or in outside facilities.  These may vary depending on the hospital or organization size.  There are also numerous nursing jobs that do not involve patient care at all.

### Labor & Delivery, Maternal Care, Neonatal Care
A favorite for many female nurses to pursue is a job in the Labor & Delivery unit.  That is perfectly cool, and lots of them love to work there.  I have not met any men who had the same desire.   I have done clinical rotations for both nursing school and my EMT program in L&D units, but never attempted to work in one.   But through my clinical rotations, I have gotten to see a number of cesarean section surgeries, along with lots of vaginal births.   It's quite an experience if you have never watched in happen in person.

The name is pretty self-explanatory.  Women go there to have babies.  The nurses care for the laboring mom, and assist the physician with the delivery.  They may also provide the immediate assessment and care of the newborn, or there may be other neonatal nurses present.  I'm not sure what the average is on that.  Pregnant mothers may also have health problems that cause complications during pregnancy, and they will be admitted to these units to have those problems treated while also monitoring the pregnancy.   Common serious health problems can suddenly be upgraded from serious to deadly in the context of pregnancy.  These nurses don't just help deliver babies.  They also specialize in many acute conditions.

In some cases, both the mother and baby remain on the L&D unit, and are both cared for by the L&D nurse.  In some hospitals they will have a separate unit where new moms and babies go, like a "postpartum unit," or "mother/baby unit." Obviously if the baby has problems, they may be taken to the neonatal ICU, which is probably more common than you think. It's not always a life and death situation. Often times the baby just requires some IV fluids or medications, or light therapy, or transfusions, etc, and this is best handled by the critical care staff who specialize in working with little bitty tiny humans. One of my own children spent a few days in the NICU just because he needed some extra IV fluid. I would be terrified to do this job. I have never tried to put an IV in a newborn baby, and I'm glad there are other nurses out there to do it.

In the similar spirit of discussing the labor-and-delivery type patients, you may come across them in the ICU occasionally. I had a few over the years, who were there because their blood pressure was so high, or some other problem. If I remember correctly, I believe they had already given birth, but were having their own postpartum problems requiring ICU care. Fortunately, in these cases, a labor and delivery nurse would come and make routine visits and assessments. If you are a mother, then you know about all the business that happens down there in the vagina neighborhood after giving birth. There is bleeding and all sorts of things I think.

On a funny note, I specifically remember one case when I had a new mother in the ICU to receive medication for dangerously high blood pressure. When I was just coming on shift, the L&D nurse was leaving after having done her assessment, so I knew that aspect of care was covered. I did all of my ICU related work, but my comfort level with L&D is very low. I wasn't really thinking about what I was saying or doing... it just sort of happened. After finishing the ICU stuff, I just sort of casually pointed at her pelvic region and asked, "Is there anything you need me to do with that vagina business and whatnot down there?" That was not very "nursing professional" of me. But she thought it was funny. I assured her that if she had a problem or concern, she could tell me and I would address any immediate emergencies and/or would call the L&D nurse to come see her, in addition to her regularly-scheduled visits.

## Pre/Post-op

Some nurses work in the surgery department or operating room (OR), and/or the pre/post-operative unit. They will prepare patients for surgery, assist with surgical procedures, and then care for patients for a limited time in the post-surgery recovery area before the patients are discharged or are admitted to a room in the hospital.

In the pre-op area, the nurse will start IV's and give medications if appropriate, and generally prep the patient in whatever way is necessary while they are still awake. Sometimes there will be teaching matters to prepare the patient for what they will experience after surgery. This may be a time when documentation is done with the patient. A common practice is to go through questions with the patient to make sure all previous procedures are documented, and note if there are special requirements or considerations.

The MRI scanner is not in the OR, but it serves as the best example. All metal must be removed from the patient, and consideration is given to all implanted devices and generally anything else that might be affected by the procedure. Even a tattoo can sometimes be a problem in the MRI. Extensive documentation is performed with the patient to cover all these issues. Perhaps there are other procedures in the OR or possibly in other procedural areas where a similar consideration might be necessary.

Another activity is for the patient, nurse, and surgeon to meet in person and jointly confirm the identification of the patient, the exact surgery that is to be done, and the exact location where it will happen. For example, if a knee replacement is to be done, the three participants may draw a big "X" or write "NO" on the knee not receiving the surgery, and write "YES" on the correct knee on which the procedure is to be done. It seems crazy, but "wrong-site" surgery mistakes still do happen. Obviously it could happen easily on an anatomical feature that has bilateral components, like two arms, and two legs. The correct arm or leg could get confused during all of the preparation and interactions by all of the staff.

Post-op is where patients go after surgery to be monitored for some period of time. This is clearly a critical step in the process, as vital signs are constantly taken, the patient is allowed to wake, mental status is assessed, and the surgical site is assessed repeatedly. Overall, close monitoring is done for any one of an endless list of possible complications. Sometimes a patient might have respiratory problems and need to be intubated again and sent to the ICU instead of going home or going to Med/Surg. Post-op nurses may also communicate with waiting family members to update on the patient's status.

There is much more to pre-op and post-op, but this gives a general taste.

## Operating Rooms

In the operating room, the nurse may or may not be "scrubbed in," meaning they have the sterile gown, gloves, and mask necessary to touch the patient or any tools being used. They will always at least have a hair cover, feet covers, and a mask when in an OR suite. It seems like in my OR rotations, the nurse was not scrubbed-in, but instead was sort of coordinating the activities in the room and doing lots of documentation. However they may also participate in aspects of the procedure in some cases. The OR techs generally manage all of the surgery tools, and an anesthesiologist takes care of the general anesthesia and monitoring of vital signs. The nurse may work with blood transfusions that are needed during the surgery, or other components of medications or special needs. I apologize that I do not have more information, but I do not want to speculate about something in which I have minimal knowledge.

Overall, just know that the job of the OR nurse goes far beyond anything I have listed here. It is a highly skilled and complex job.

I have never worked OR or Recovery. Like everything else, some nurses love it and make a career out of it. Others might get tired of it quickly. It's totally up to the individual.

**Interventional Radiology**

Interventional Radiology (IR) is a specialty unit that performs procedures similar to surgery, but the patient is generally not under complete sedation. Further, these procedures are done using a variety of imaging tools, like x-ray or CT scanners. The interventional radiologist will do all sorts of procedures while watching the actions inside the body via imaging. They have something called fluoroscopy, which looks like a moving x-ray. So, a live x-ray video is playing in front of the physician, and he uses it to guide his actions inside the body. It's really a pretty cool place, and there are lots of interesting procedures to see.

Like surgery, patient interactions are brief. There is the pre-op phase where the nurse preps the patient for the procedure, then as the procedure happens the nurse will administer sedation/pain medication and/or monitor vitals signs and/or assist the physician with the procedure itself. These procedures may or may not have an anesthesiologist, but that just depends on the nature of the case. If there is no anesthesiologist present, then the nurse is managing sedation and monitoring the patient.

Then the patient will be monitored in a post-op manner, like that described above, for some short period of time before being discharged or sent back up to a hospital room. So, if you like working with procedures, and not really having to get involved with the normal aspects of patient care in a hospital unit, this can be a really fun and exciting job to have. I have known some nurses who had a lot of fun working in this area, and had a new-found joy in their work after feeling burned out from an inpatient unit.

**Cardiac Catheterization Lab (Cath Lab)**

Cath lab is another exciting procedural unit in which a nurse may work. It is similar to interventional radiology, except all of the procedures are related to the heart and its surrounding structures, and other aspects of the blood vessels throughout the body. So, when a patient is having an active heart attack, they are often times rushed into the cath lab, where the interventional cardiologist will use imaging (like in IR) to guide his or her work. They will insert catheters into the large veins and arteries, and thread them up into the heart. They can then deposit radiopaque dye, which shows up on the x-ray, and so the physician can see how the blood is flowing through the coronary arteries. Once the blockages are located, they can thread a tiny catheter into those arteries around the heart, inflate a balloon to open up the blockage, and then deploy a stent to hold the artery open. It is really awesome to see this done.

They will also do routine scheduled heart catheterizations for various diagnostic purposes, or possibly for placement of things like pacemakers. Nurses, like in interventional radiology, will prep patients, assist with the procedures, administer medications, manage sedation, monitor the patient during the procedure, and then provide temporary post-operative care before the patient is discharged or admitted to a hospital room.

IR and cath lab staff are on call a lot, as they will be emergently called in at any time of the night to do a an emergent procedure (especially cath lab for heart attacks). I have known lots of cath lab nurses, and they all love what they do. I considered moving to the cath lab, and actually had an offer, but opted to take the ICU charge nurse position instead.

Now, I could be totally wrong about this, but I have always felt like interventional radiology and cath lab nurses, while getting to do an exciting job, lack much of the autonomy that ICU nurses have. A physician is present during the entire procedure, and so their need for making life-and-death decisions on their own may be limited. I also found this to be true in my emergency department experience, as while the ER physician may not be in each room continuously, they are on the unit and immediately available to any nurse at any time for any emergency.

Again, I mean no disrespect towards any of these nurses. They are highly experienced and skilled at what they do, and I could not do their job for them without a great deal of training. So I do not wish to imply my ICU experience is any better. It is just different. I enjoy my ICU autonomy. In the procedural areas and ER, the workflow is just different, the patient interactions are different, and the unexpected nature of the processes are different, so the constant presence of a physician counterbalances these variable. In the ICU, we are in a very controlled environment, and so successful autonomy comes easier.

**Gastroenterology Lab (or "GI Lab")**
This procedural area is where all sorts of tasks related to the digestive system are done. This includes things like a "colonoscopy," during which long tube with a camera is inserted into the rectum and threaded through the large intestine. Another is the "esophagogastroduodenoscopy"

(EGD), in which the long tube with a camera is inserted through the mouth and down the esophagus to see the inside of the stomach and the first part of the small intestines. The "esophageal (or endoscopic) retrograde cholangio-pancreatography" (ERCP) involves sending at tube with a camera far enough down through the stomach and into the small intestines, so that the gall bladder and ducts to the liver and pancreas can be visualized.

These tubes with cameras also have a set of tools built in that can perform various tasks. The gastroenterologist might be able to deploy a clamp over an area of bleeding, or directly inject epinephrine into the spot to constrict the blood vessels, both in an attempt to stop the flow of blood. A polyp or growth or other abnormality may be found and a sample can be removed for testing, or the whole growth or polyp removed. In the case of the ERCP, a blocked bile duct (gall stones) near the gallbladder and liver can be opened. Other structural abnormalities may be examined or surgically manipulated.

Patients in these procedures are usually not under full general anesthesia, but will be under deep sedation, which may be performed and/or monitored by a nurse or another physician, depending on the types of drugs used. The nurse will also perform continuous monitoring of the patient and his or her vital signs, etc while the physician focuses only on the procedure. A technician or nurse may also assist the physician with the equipment and procedure.

**Nursing Education**

Working in nursing education can be done in several ways. The most obvious is teaching at a nursing school and/or teaching and monitoring students during clinical rotations. This may require a BSN to teach LPN students, or a master's degree in nursing to teach RN students. If you want to teach BSN students, I believe a doctoral degree is required. You would have to check with the local nursing schools on these requirements. They may vary from place to place. Also, there may be jobs where you work as a clinical instructor, but are not the primary teacher/professor/instructor for the students, and so a lesser degree may be allowed. I believe that some instructors only teach in the classroom, while others only do the clinical rotations, and some instructors will do both. Again, you would have to check with your local schools.

I am not sure how well teaching pays. But, your work schedule will mirror that of the school schedules, meaning holidays, weekends, and time between semesters (or even the entire summer in some cases) will be off. So, theoretically, it may break down that your overall annual salary is less than a floor nurse. But perhaps when considering the actual hours worked, and the amount of time during the year when no work is happening, but paychecks are still coming, maybe the pay is actually really good in comparison. And, with so much time off on weekends, between semesters, and maybe even during and entire summer, the nursing instructor may pick up extra work.

One of my LPN nursing school instructors would pick up a shift here and there at the hospital where I worked, and I would occasionally work with him on the unit (when I was a CNA). That felt strange at first. One day in class you have to call him Mr. Doe. And then later that same night at work you call him John. The point is that many full-time nursing instructors will also pick up hospital shifts on the weekends to keep their skills sharp and keep their foot in the door in case they want to stop teaching and come back to the hospital.

The next nursing education opportunity is within a hospital. Large hospitals usually have an entire nursing education department, with some number of RN's and a unit director or manager. They may or may not be attached to human resources. In my hospital they were a fully independent department. In addition to all of the RN's that staffed the department, a number of additional RN's are present as representatives of their specific unit in the hospital. So, for example, we had a position in the ICU called "ICU Nurse Educator." This nurse worked with the unit and with the education department to manage all things education-related on their specific unit. The nurse educators and education department are jointly charged with training new nurses, and managing credentials of existing nurses. In the nursing world, especially in hospitals, nurses must be tested or "checked-off" each year on many of the skills they regularly perform. And, all nurses must have a certain number of qualified continuing-education units, or CEU's each year in order to keep their license in good standing with the state. The hospital may require that each nurse also register their CEU's with the education department, to ensure licenses are not in jeopardy, and may require certain CEU's to be completed, such as stroke or heart attack protocols. In the ICU, this list of skills is particularly high, considering all of the advanced equipment, decision-making, and skills performed.

The education department, and specifically the unit nurse educator, will spend countless hours observing nurses performing certain skills in order to sign off on their competency. Some nurses, once checked-off, may then have the power to check-off other nurses. In my department, that usually meant the charge nurses were checked-off first, and then they also had the ability to check-off other staff nurses.

This process can be long and cumbersome, as nurses must often wait for an opportunity to arise to perform a specific skill while under observation. Nurses will have to cooperate to get opportunities to do all skills within a given time period of a month (give or take). You will hear nurses asking around if they can do skills on other nurses' patients, or some nurses asking if anyone needs to come do a specific skill on their patient.

Some skills may require attendance to a re-certification class, along with a test. The most common example of this is the BLS (Basic Life Support) certification all nurses in the hospital must have, and the ACLS (Advanced Cardiac Life Support) certification, which ER and ICU nurses must get. Pediatric units may require their nurses to get PALS (Pediatric Advanced Life Support), and ER nurses may have certain trauma certifications, along with the PALS, as they see all ages of patients. BLS, ACLS, PALS, and certain trauma certifications each will involve one or two full days of classes and skills practice. The more advanced of the certifications, like ACLS, will usually take something like 16 hours of work, distributed between two full days. The life-support classes may be taught by nursing educator staff, or also by ER or ICU nurses who have been qualified to do so with additional certifications. Life support training is just one example. There are many other possible classes depending on the unit. All hours spent in these classes in the hospital were on-the-clock paid time.

The periods when all of the hospital-wide check-offs are being completed are very hectic time for education staff, for obvious reasons. They have to process every individual nurse in the hospital, and ensure that each has completed their unit-specific or job-specific educational requirements, along with CEU's and skills check-offs.

Another major aspect of the nurse educator staff, both on the unit and departmentally, is to work with all new nurses who join the hospital team. From the new baby nurses, all the way up to the most experienced veteran nurses, all staff will generally enjoy an orientation period before they are turned loose to work independently. For the new graduate nurses, especially in the higher acuity units like ER or ICU, they will go through a "nurse internship," which may last up to six months. During the internship, they will spend every shift working with and/or under the supervision of an experienced preceptor on the unit. Preceptors are just staff who are willing to train new nurses. Some nurses don't like doing it. Some do. I loved doing it. The preceptor assignment may be kept constant, so the new nurses's schedule will mirror the preceptor's schedule, and they will work together every shift for weeks or months.

In our hospital, the nurse interns, in addition to working shifts with a preceptor, would attend all necessary classes for advanced skills and certifications needed, and would spend time completing the required CEU's for the hospital. They may also spend classroom time learning the computer system, and go through days of general hospital orientation (which is done by all staff, including business and non-medical people) to learn about the employment policies and employee handbook, etc. They may do one shift in each other department as an observer in order to understand how that department works in relation to their own. I got to do this, and it was just like doing clinical rotations again. They may have to take tests on medications and drug dosing calculations, along with scenario-based testing.

In our emergency department, I think the new nurses spent additional time in the Neonatal ICU in order to get extra training on working with the little bitty tiny humans. And, our ER interns would do at least one "ride-out" with an ambulance crew for a 12-hour shift.

During the internship, which once again may last up to six months, there will be follow-up interviews with unit directors and/or managers to discuss progress, along with preceptors and other staff nurses.

I have always thought nursing education is cool. If I had finished my master's degree, I was actually considering teaching. In the hospital-based education departments, the nurse educators must keep their skills up so they can train and assess the other nurses. So it is one possible way to get to do "nursing stuff," but not really have to take care of patients.

## Business

I have never worked in the capacity of an "office nurse." Some nurses will work jobs that involve absolutely no clinical or hands-on work with patients, and generally have no patient contact at all. They may wear suites or other traditional business attire, as opposed to scrubs. I don't know a lot about these jobs, except that they exist. This may involve working with the billing department to interpret medical documentation for appropriate charges, or reviewing medical documentation to audit for specific types of abnormalities. There was one of these type nurses in the nursing home in which I worked, and I know there were some in the hospital. I will not pretend to know much more about them. But I do know their job is important.

## Case-Specific Specialists

This is a broad category. In my hospital system, we had positions called CHF Coordinator, Chest Pain/STEMI Coordinator, Stroke Coordinator, Quality Coordinator, Risk Coordinator, Infection Control Coordinator, and Code Coordinator. There may have been more. These are just the ones I can remember at the moment. Some of these were just a single nurse, and some were an entire department in the hospital system.

The CHF, Chest Pain/STEMI, and Stroke Coordinators are essentially the nurses who have an involvement in all of these sorts of cases in the hospital. Not hands-on with the patient, but in a capacity to ensure compliance with all state and oversight agency requirements, and compliance with hospital policies and procedures. There are endless expectations from various state agencies and hospital credentialing organizations.

For example, in terms of the Chest Pain/STEMI Coordinator, the word "STEMI" stands for "S-T Elevation Myocardial Infarction," which is a complicated way to say "a big heart attack." There are different types of heart attacks. This particular one is the most serious, and results in emergent transfer to the cath lab, or into surgery if appropriate. The exact way in which a chest pain or STEMI case is handled will be directed by complex sets of algorithms and standards set by hospital policy. This will include the amount of time to pass before and during certain interventions. It will guide the types of medications a physician will order before, during, and after interventions. It will require certain actions by the nurse, such as specific documentation standards, nurse-patient education, and emergency response actions.

Hospitals will generally have certifications and designations about what type of patient they can handle. These case-specific nurses will work with the physicians, emergency department, inpatient units, procedural departments, management, and various committees to ensure compliance with requirements necessary to obtain or maintain a certification.

I will dedicate a chapter later to discussing these case experts, the job they do, how it relates to hospital policies and procedures, and how it directly affects the work of each individual nurse. You will find that this leads into a much broader discussion about "best practices," audits, nursing and physician documentation, and the relationship between the hospital and the various oversight and licensing agencies.

## Outside Companies, Support, Sales

Nurses or technicians representing certain device companies will monitor and manage the usage of some devices. Examples of this would be the nurse or tech who works for the company that makes a type of pacemaker. These nurses or technicians will be present when the device is surgically implanted, and will do their own sets of assessments and testing to know it is working accurately. They may perform later testing or assessment on the patient in the days following the procedure. They may also provide formal training classes to hospital staff, or short education in-services on each unit, regarding existing or new devices and skills related to care, upkeep, maintenance, and use. There are countless different nurses and technicians like this.

In the ICU, we had phone and pager numbers for on-call staff representing each piece of specialized equipment and the company that manufactures it. If we had a problem with an intra-aortic balloon pump during the night, we would page the balloon pump guy (usually an RN) from the balloon pump company, and he would provide over-the-phone technical support, and in some cases would actually come into the hospital to provide assistance or maintenance.

Some nurses will work in sales, either while also doing the above-listed technical and educational support, or on its own. Device companies are continuously changing, updating, and inventing new equipment. This goes for everything from the type of bandage we put over a wound, to the hospital bed, to the most highly specialized and advanced machinery. Sales staff from these companies will visit hospital leadership and staff to essentially sell their equipment.

This may or may not involve a great deal of travel, a company car, an expense account, treating hospital staff to dinner, giving presentations to hospital committees, and/or negotiating order sizes and pricing. There are tons of medical supply companies out there competing with each other. Each want us to use their specific ointment, or dressing, or transfer device, or bed, or IV pump, or life-support machine. And hospitals will frequently make changes in suppliers and/or equipment, meaning a completely different line of wound-care supplies will suddenly appear in the supply room.

Then, a nurse or technician from that company will visit all the departments to educate and even "check-off" skills for nurses on the new tools. In the case of something more complicated than wound dressings, they will hold a series of classes over the course of a few weeks to make sure every applicable staff member receives appropriate training.

## Case Management, Social Worker, Social and Charity Programs

Case Managers assist in planning post-discharge care for a patient, such as organizing nursing home placement or organizing home health coverage when a patient is being discharged home, or working out the details if a patient needs to be transferred to another facility. They assess for specific patient needs, and help the healthcare team provide seamless continuity of care. Some patients may have a complicated home situation, in which they were abused or otherwise unsafe, and work must be done to ensure a safe disposition upon discharge from the hospital. Patients may have trouble affording medications, meaning work must be done to help them plan ahead for this problem before they go home. This may even involve the case manager working with the physician to change prescriptions if needed and possible.

Many patients will have advanced directives, or medical powers of attorney, in which they legally have instructed as to how their care will be handled and/or who will be allowed to make decisions for them if they are unable to speak for themselves (comatose, confused, any sort of altered mental status). I would generally refer to case management anybody who wanted to inquire about these things. I am not a lawyer, and staff is limited to only direct care medical personnel at night, so I would write an order to case management to come in the next day to assist with this in whatever way was necessary. Many times, case management was my go-to resource if something non-medical or unrelated to the current medical care was of concern, and assistance was needed.

Hospitals do not just discharge a patient and wheel them out the front door with no plan in place for how they will be cared for. For the general otherwise healthy and competent person who can go home and continue with normal life, this process is easy, and usually just involves helping them schedule followup appointments. When the vulnerable population is involved (homeless, financial insufficiency to afford care/medications, abusive or unsafe home environment, patient not mentally competent to make decisions for themselves, patients with no support structure outside the hospital, patients needing to go to a nursing home or a rehabilitation facility, etc), case management will help to ensure a plan is in place for these people prior to discharge.

I love case managers, because they do a lot of the jobs I don't want to do, but that need to be done. I mentioned in my story early in the book about loving that I just do medical stuff. I no longer have to deal with the company's, or somebody else's money, or other issues unrelated to the medical problem in front of me. All aspects of the organization are important. I just don't want to do certain parts myself. And the case manager work falls into that category of "that's somebody else's job." And, when I was on duty at night, I had no access to any "office people" anyway, so I used to just order case manager consultations all the time.

Patient 1: "I don't have insurance and I'm not sure how I'm going to pay..."

Me: "Bam! case manager consult."

Patient 2: "I can't drive anymore so I don't know how I will get to..."

Me: "Bam! case manager consult."
Patient 3: "My rent is going to be a month behind when I get home so..."
Me: "Bam! case manager consult."
Patient 4: "I have questions about doing a power of attorney for..."
Me: "Bam! case manager consult."
Patient 5: "I am concerned about the side effects of metoprolol when I get home.
Me: "Bam!.... well, metoprolol is a beta blocker, which means it can both lower heart rate and blood pressure. So the main initial concern is symptoms related to that. Like, if you stand up too fast you might get dizzy...
Patient 6: "I don't like the nursing home where I live..."
Me: "Bam! case manager consult."

Obviously, the work of the case manager is super important, and the system would break down without them. For some, it is their calling to take on these sorts of challenge. To make sure a patient can access the medications they need, to make sure the battered and abused wife has a safe place to go away from their aggressor, to make sure a child in a questionable household is safe, to make sure a hostile family dynamic will not harm the patient, to make sure each patient has a safe place to live after discharge. To provide power to the powerless, strength to the weak, hope to the hopeless, help to the helpless, safety to the vulnerable, dignity to the exposed, and access to resources for those who society might otherwise let fall through the cracks (one might say their job is very inspiring!).

In some less-developed countries, the elderly and sick are left on the street to die, as they have no one to take care of them, and no social system is in place to help them. We don't do things like that in the USA. And regardless of your political affiliation and personal opinions on social programs like welfare, food stamps, Medicaid, Medicare, and social security, we, as a medical community, like to give every single patient a fighting chance once they leave the hospital.

You will check your own facility's policies and procedures when it comes to ordering case manager consults, and knowing exactly what they do.

I have a quick funny story. When I was working in the nursing home, an older man wandered in. He was dirty and disheveled. He looked physically stable overall, but it was clear that he had nothing and nobody. I didn't hear his story, but I think he had either been living on the street, or was about to live on the street as his outside family support system had come apart. He came in because he was tired and didn't feel good, and he didn't know where to go. He thought we might be a doctor's office, considering the name on the building. When he looked medically stable, we just called the social worker out of her office and handed him off to her. When I came back the next day, he was living there. I guess they got him set up with Medicaid or something. I don't even know. They may have taken him on as a charity case (which is a real type of program). I was just pleased to see him safe and secure. How cool is that!?!

We had cases in the ICU (frequently) where a patient had been sick for a long time, and had become medically fragile, and had even become dependent on a ventilator. They have no money or insurance. They can't go to a nursing home under Medicaid, as they are too medically compromised. They need to go to a long-term acute care facility. Obviously, no outside facility wants to accept somebody who they know will not pay for their care. However, most of these facilities have some sort of charity program in place, where they have a designated number of beds reserved for these exact sorts of cases. So, in some of our ICU patients, they ended up spending extra weeks or even months just living in our ICU on their ventilator, until a case manager finally found a charity bed that could take them.  Did the hospital get paid for that person's long hospitalization and critical care?  Obviously not.  But the system is set up that we don't just throw a person onto the street because they can't pay.

I am not going to get all political here.  But social programs, or "socialist" programs as some political persuasions like to call them (looking at you red states), really are critically important for our vulnerable population.  I will not pretend I have the knowledge or expertise to pass judgement on the politics of social programs.  That is super complicated stuff.  If you, dear reader, think you know enough about them to pass judgement and have a solid political opinion, I would suggest you do an internet search for the term: "Dunning-Kruger Effect."  Then, seriously assess what your level of knowledge is, and how that realistically aligns with your claimed confidence in said knowledge.  (Sorry, that is a bit of a tangent from the discussion).  Anyway, as a medical professional, I see where social programs are the most critical, and where they legitimately save lives. And I am personally comforted to know that there is a safety net down there if I ever topple off my privileged American middle-class pedestal and am no longer able to take care of myself.

Case managers might be staffed by RN's or Licensed Social Workers.

## Management/Leadership

As mentioned other places in this book, there is always some sort of management hierarchy within a nursing department.  The size and nature of this structure can vary greatly depending mainly on the size of a hospital and specific department.

For example, I spent some time in a sort of private-duty home health scenario that was paid for by a special program under Medicaid (I think), but don't quote me on that. As I have said, I loved the fact that my job in nursing had nothing to do with from whence the money came, nor where it went, as long as it just went into my paycheck, and my only job was to do medical stuff! In this setup, I basically worked independently, and was the "RN Supervisor" for the case. Of course the physicians and specialists for the kid wrote all medication and treatment orders, etc. I was not making up my own orders. However, I did not really have a boss to report to, as I was directly employed by the parents of the patient. They had to do evaluations and paperwork on me to send to the other money outfit, whatever it was, but I reported to them. When the parents hired an LPN and a CNA to work some with the patient when I was not on duty, I acted as their "supervisor." It may vary from state to state what the exact rules are, but generally the LPN/LVN is required to function under, and report to, an RN supervisor of some sort.

Within the very large hospital, where I worked, the system was more complicated. A "Chief Nursing Officer" (CNO) was the ultimate authority at the top, and worked with the other top brass of the company, the chief executive officer, chief medical officer, chief finance officer, etc. I don't know what a CNO gets paid. One would assume it is better than what a floor nurse makes! The CNO is responsible for all nursing activity in the whole hospital, and sometimes in multiple hospitals when smaller facilities are connected or nearby. There might be assistant CNO's too.

From my experience, the next level down was generally the departmental directors. Sometimes these positions would cover only one large unit, or possibly multiple units similar or connected to one another. On my Med/Surg unit, we had a director that was responsible for three units total.

Underneath the director was the "unit manager." Each unit manager was responsible for one single "unit" or floor or otherwise smaller subsection of the hospital.

The unit managers were the most hands-on leadership for the unit, and would be the most common leadership position with which floor nurses would interact during day-to-day business on the unit, although the director would be present occasionally. Managers were often still safely tucked away in an office, and very rarely had patient interactions beyond addressing certain complaints or problems, or doing routine courtesy visits to patients and families in the room. However, they may sometimes emerge from their offices and help (temporarily) with patient care if things are overly-busy, or the staff is terribly short. They are generally available to the nurses for anything needed above the pay-grade of the charge nurse.

A series of charge nurses would be on staff, under the manager, to ultimately run the hands-on patient care operations on the unit. CNO's, directors, and managers are commonly daytime jobs, and may remain on call for major hospital-wide emergencies, but would generally sleep well each night. Charge nurses were the ones to be ever-present, continuously managing each functional staff member on the unit under the nursing structure (RN's, LPN's, CNA's, and nursing students). The hospital can run without the continuous presence of CNO's, directors, and managers (like weekends and nights). But a charge nurse must always be on duty, even if it meant having a staff RN step up and do the job occasionally when a regular charge nurse calls in sick. In fact, that was how I made my way into charging.

Daytime charge nurse: "Brett, we don't have a charge nurse tonight. You will be doing the job."

Me: "Uh, okay, I will do my best..." (With terrified look on face)

I worked as a fill-in charge occasionally when a regular one was not available, and this eventually led to the promotion to full permanent charge nurse. (That very first shift was pretty rocky, but I survived, as did all of the other nurses and patients)

In some really large units, like the Level I Trauma Center, there were also a few "team leaders," which may work as a sort of back-up for a specific subset of nurses or "pods" in the unit, and will be the liaison between the staff nurses nurses and the charge nurse.

Another leadership position of great importance is the "hospital supervisor," also often called "house supervisor." The hospital supervisors report directly to the CNO or assistant CNO, but otherwise do not intermix with the unit leadership the same way. Their rank is about equivalent to a unit director, but they have hospital-wide responsibility in the day-to-day operations related directly to patient care. The hospital supervisor is the liaison that coordinates efforts between hospital units, along with other functions. They help organize the logistics for moving patients between units and procedures, help sort out problems between units, and interact with other hospitals, facilities, ambulance services, helicopter services, etc to coordinate patient movement.

They will often manage staffing for the whole hospital from one shift to the next. If one unit is overstaffed, and another understaffed, they would work with the charge nurses to make sure all units had the necessary resources. If certain teams need to be called in emergently during the night (like cath lab), they often will perform those communications and coordinate with those teams to ensure all resources are in place. Although they rank the same as unit directors, they are functionally more like charge nurses, in that there is one on duty at all times, no matter what. But, they still do outrank the charge nurse.

Clearly, during the day, there is a full cadre of nursing leaders and managers. At night the staffing is very thin. On a given night when I was charge nurse in the ICU, the highest ranking nursing official in the building was the hospital supervisor. Each inpatient unit had a charge nurse. So, each charge nurse reports to the hospital supervisor. In an extreme situation or problem, the hospital supervisor may call the CNO or a unit director at home. But that was rare. So, at night, hospital supervisor is in charge of nursing, charge nurses are in charge of the units.

As the ICU charge nurse, I was the highest level and most skilled hands-on nurse in the hospital. The ICU charge nurse and the hospital supervisor jointly respond to all emergencies. The hospital supervisor works to coordinate the process, like transferring the patient to the ICU or to another facility. Meanwhile, the ICU charge nurse is directing the hands-on care of the patient.

Of course, I must acknowledge the presence of the highly skilled nurses of the ER. However, I don't count them in any of these discussions, because they didn't respond to anything in the hospital. They are almost like their own separate facility within the same building. The ER doctor would come to a code-blue in order to intubate the patient, but that was the extent of the ER's involvement, so I generally leave them out of the inpatient functions.

It can be a little confusing. So don't worry too much. You will start as a staff nurse and figure the rest out later. Different positions may require different education levels. And you may find yourself at a facility that is totally different from my experience.

## Advanced Practice Nurse

The "advanced practice nurse" (APN) is sort of a generic term for a nurse who has obtained education, license, and/or certification to perform in a higher level scope of practice. There are many opportunities for the APN beyond normal clinical nursing work. I have discussed some of this already in the nursing school and licenses chapter of the book.

One of the more commonly recognized positions is the "Nurse Practitioner" (NP). These professionals have all of the components of being an RN, but have an additional degree (masters or doctorate), along with having completed certain clinical rotation requirements, and having passed specific state licensing exams. They, like physicians, have the authority to make medical diagnoses and prescribe medications (although with limitations). They may also have more advanced clinical skills beyond what RN's are allowed to do. We see lots of these positions in nursing homes, doctors offices (regular or specialized), hospitals (assisting a physician), and walk-in clinics.

They may also work with a specialty physician, or just for the hospital, in a capacity where they focus on one type of patient. For example, in the large hospital, there was an advanced practice nurse who worked for pulmonology, and would visit and monitor all patients in the hospital who had a tracheostomy. Even if the patient was not being seen by pulmonology, this nurse would visit and evaluate and communicate with the staff nurses about any problems or needs. If we admitted a patient to the hospital who had a trach, we would just write a referral or consult order for the "trach nurse." She would come around during normal business hours and see the patient once a day. If a patient in the hospital had a new trach and was to be discharged, she would work with them to help prepare for their self-care at home.

One of my fellow charge nurses in the ICU completed his family nurse practitioner program, and became licensed. He left the ICU and went to work in the pain clinic. I don't know how much he did with procedures, but I'm sure a lot of his job was seeing patients in routine appointments and renewing prescriptions. Many (or most, or maybe all) chronic pain patients who are on continuous opiate pain medications are seen monthly in the pain clinic. Their prescriptions will only be renewed for one month at a time, and they must make these appearances. They will even be drug tested periodically to make sure the drug they are being prescribed is in their system (they are taking it and not selling it, etc) and that there are no other drugs present.

In modern times, many patients never see an actual doctor when they have appointments at their family practice clinic, or when they go to a walk-in clinic. They see a nurse practitioner. In some ER's there may be a nurse practitioner on duty who sees all of the low-acuity stuff, like sore throats, freeing up the ER physicians to focus on the more complex cases. In some places nurse practitioners even own their own independent medical practice, like a family-care clinic. They still have oversight by higher medical authority, a physician I presume, but I do not know how all that works. If you become a practitioner and open your own clinic one day, you will figure that out.

Their pay is generally better than RN floor nurse pay, but they are not getting rich.

You would have to check with your state's board of nursing to fully define the exact licenses, specializations, and scopes of practice.

The "certified registered nurse anesthetist" (CRNA) is a highly favorable position, with substantial earning potential. A CRNA may be the highest paid job a person can get in nursing, or at least compete with a CNO. I have met a few physicians over the years who actually say they wish they would have done CRNA instead of medical school.

The CRNA is a highly specialized position within the anesthesia realm. They work with and under physician anesthesiologists, and can perform many of the same functions. For example, they can manage a patient under general anesthesia during a surgery, a job normally reserved for the anesthesiologists. They will do lots of lower-level procedural sedation as well. They mostly work in procedural areas, like surgery. They may also perform skills like placement of catheters for epidural pain medications (like the epidural a laboring mother gets while giving birth).

This certification requires a masters or doctorate, depending on the school and state, along with having completed a rigorous and challenging couple or few years of school work that likely rivals the intensity of medical school. These schools are highly competitive to get into, and require a heavy time and energy investment, but the resulting jobs are phenomenal. Their earning potential may rival many physicians.

**Nursing Informatics**

This is an interesting and rapidly growing aspect of the nursing world. With the emergence and requirements of electronic documentation and medical record systems, there are now unimaginably complex computer programs, which are designed to manage all of the business that flows through an organization, from the nurses writing their notes, the physician writing orders, the pharmacy processing medications, the labs and radiology imaging/testing/results, to the upper leadership managing budgets and statistical information and the billing department handling the money.

With these programs come large tech companies with armies of computer programmers, and hardware specialists, and engineers, etc. And, there is a small army of nurses to manage the clinical and medical aspect of system design, and in managing the real-life application of the systems, within the tech company itself. Medicine is already intolerably complicated. So now if you want to take that limitless complexity, and build it into algorithms and programs and systems, which are user friendly enough for all hospital staff, from the housekeeper up to the CNO, and work appropriately with numerous different departments and specializations, clinical to technical to financial, a whole new specialization in the technical and medical world has been born.

During the time I was working in the large hospital organization, they overhauled the limited computer system we had, along with the paper charts, and consolidated it all into a new electronic medical program, which took years from start to finish. Really, it may have been up to five years or more for the whole transition. An outside tech company designed the system, and then worked with us to make it "fit" into our hospital. It was the full-time job of an entire new department in the hospital, staffed by numerous RN's and hospital IT folks, to work on this transition. And, that was just in the planning and design phase for a few years. When the program showed up in our computers, running parallel to our older system, the amount of meetings, training classes, testing groups, and feedback processes was quite unbelievable. Each person in the hospital system who would use the system (several large hospitals, several small hospitals, countless clinics out in the communities, a new hospital being built, etc, doctors, nurses, money people, etc) had to take anywhere from two to five half-day classes to learn the new system. That must have cost many millions of dollars just for the staff to sit in classes while on the clock, outside of their normal productive work time.

The large entirely new department was active in our hospital system for years, staffed with lots of nurses and computer people, with its own management structure, just to prepare for the program to arrive. Then once it arrived, the department spent another year working through implementation, feedback, fixes, more meetings, committees.... I don't know how many millions were spent just to get the program, but many more had to be spent to smoothly transition our system to it.

Ultimately, electronic medical records systems create an unimaginably large new business sector in both the healthcare and technology economies.

So, if you are a sort of mix of a nurse and a computer nerd, something like this may be perfect for you if you get tired of clinical work!

## Clinics

Clinics are fairly self-explanatory, although there are some variations. A traditional doctor's office, like a family medicine physician, will have a nurse who will take patients back, take vitals and measurements, review medications and medical history and allergies, administer any ordered medications, and assist with many other aspects of paperwork, phone communications with patients, and office routines.

Some other clinics are very specialized. For example, a dialysis clinic is where dialysis patients go from home two or three days a week to be connected to the dialysis machine for several hours. There are pain management clinics, coumadin clinics, neurology clinics, CHF clinics, and cardiology clinics, just to name a few. There are many more. Different clinics may have nurses performing or assisting in specific procedures. For example, the physician in a pain clinic may administer steroid injections into various joints or into the spine, and much of this may be done under x-ray guidance. The skill level for nurses in these specialized clinics is far higher than that of the nurse in a family practice clinic.

Many clinics staff LPN's still, and probably will for the foreseeable future. An RN license may be required for some of the more advanced specialty clinics when procedures are involved.

## Hospice/Palliative Care

"Palliative care" basically means a healthcare model that focuses on a goal of comfort rather than a goal of cure. Hospice is an organization that manages these palliative care patients. I'll talk extensively about death and the dying process later. But, for now, many patients who are terminally ill and imminently approaching death will choose to be "made comfortable." So, some or all curative efforts may be stopped (antibiotics, diabetes management, dialysis, surgeries, constant vital signs, life support machines, invasive/painful devices, etc). Instead, they'll have very generous orders for pain and anxiety medications. They'll avoid painful treatments and procedures. They may have other treatments or medications available to promote comfort, which might not normally be used on a traditional patient. Many will have a continuous IV infusion of an opiate, like morphine or fentanyl or hydromorphone, and/or an anxiety medicine, like lorazepam or midazolam. Opiate medications are obviously great for pain control, but they also have the effect of suppressing the respiratory drive. So, if a patient is dying of lung disease, and feels like he or she is suffocating, an opiate basically takes away the desire to breath. So they can stop breathing, or fail to breathe sufficiently, and it doesn't hurt.

I won't try to discuss all the details here. Basically all efforts are directed at the patient being comfortable until he or she dies, with the understanding that these interventions may speed up the dying process. It's NOT the same thing as assisted suicide. Assisted suicide is an intervention that directly causes death, regardless of the patient's condition. Palliative care provides comfort medications so the patient doesn't hurt. Because they don't hurt, they may not fight as hard to breath, for example. So they may expire sooner. However, they're still dying from a physiological cause that would immanently bring death, with or without the comfort medications. They are still dying from natural causes. We are just taking away the pain while they do.

**Psychiatric Nursing**

Nurses may work in psychiatric or drug rehabilitation facilities. This is pretty self explanatory. It's nursing, with a primary population of patients facing mental health and/or substance abuse problems. These could be units in a hospital that are actually locked down, so patients are not able to leave. Or it could be an outside facility where all patients are there voluntarily to deal with addiction. Or it could be a state hospital or other mental health facility that deals in dangerous patients, or those who have been committed.

We saw lots of patients come through the ER and the ICU who had made some attempt at suicide. Most often it was an intentional overdose. These folks would be put under an order of emergency detention, which meant they are not free to leave the hospital. Once it's time for discharge, they are taken by law enforcement to a psychiatric hospital for treatment (against their will). Most cooperated fully and caused no trouble about getting treatment.

**Prisons and Jails**

There are hundreds of thousands of jail and prison inmates in the United States. Clearly, they are not all healthy. And, even those who are healthy may have a basic blood pressure or cholesterol medication, or psychiatric medication like an antidepressant or anti-anxiety medication, or something else specialized like a seizure medication. Some might need insulin injections multiple times each day. In some cases a prisoner may have more advanced medical needs, perhaps something that would normally have them in a nursing home, or they may require more advanced treatments like dialysis. Some prisons have specialized units for those folks. Some types of facilities may be a sort of fully functional hospital housed within a prison. Managing the medication and medical needs of the prison and jail population is a serious business in healthcare.

Prisons may have a staff of nurses who do routine

143

assessments on all inmates in the facility upon arrival, or when a complaint is had. They also provide treatments and administer medications, like any other nurse. Many large prisons have physicians and dentists on staff, along with a large fully-functional pharmacy. Prisoners will see physicians for minor complaints, or will have regular appointments with a physician for monitoring of a specific disease process, medication, or treatment.

Basically, you must remember that the massive prison population is no different from the general population in our country. Many will have medical problems, and just because they are in prison does not mean they will not have their medical needs covered or receive their medications. Nursing in a prison is just like nursing in other family practice clinic, long-term care units, and specialized treatment area. The patients are just prisoners instead of free people.

The job does not come without risks, obviously. Dealing with mental illness or those prone to violence can be a legitimate concern. But the medical staff are pretty well protected and very few incidents actually occur. Some nurses may just not want to be exposed to that environment. Other nurses may love prison nursing because they feel like they are helping people get their lives back together and stay healthy while they are rehabilitated for societal reentry. It is a special population for sure.

It's not exactly the same thing, but nurses will often take care of prison or jail inmates in the regular hospital as well. I have done it many times in the ER, Med/Surg unit, and the ICU. If a patient has chest pain or some other medical condition at a local jail, they will be shackled up and brought to the hospital either by the jail staff or by ambulance. They will be treated just like any other patient, however they will be in handcuffs and leg shackles at all times, and two armed guards will always be present in these cases. There is usually one that stays in the room, and one that sits out in the hall. I have never had a safety concern related to these situations. I have always found the patients to be polite, kind, and thankful for the care and treatment. They are not monsters. They are people. They have made bad choices at some point in life. But they are still people and are still deserving of the same patience, compassion, care, and dignity owed to any other person.

It is not the nurse's job to be mean, or stand-offish, or short, or abrupt, or unfriendly, or overly unemotional, or aggressively self-protective with these people. You don't need to stand at a distance and act like you are afraid to touch them or outwardly show that you are offended by their presence. It is not your job to participate in their punishment. The jails or prisons are already punishing them for their mistakes. You do not need to help.

If you really want to be kind-hearted and angelic, consider going the extra mile to be friendly and accommodating. Bring them coffee and snacks (if they are allowed to have them). Offer to bring coffee to the guards. Make the room a friendly environment. Do not ask them what they did. And if they try to talk about it, do not enter into a discussion. But, you will find that they will generally not want to talk much, and rarely would offer any personal information.

Speak kindly to them. Be patient with them. Give them their medications on time, and keep up with their pain medications, or anything else that provides comfort. I have seen nurses sit at the nurse station, not really doing anything important, and they owe a dose of pain medication to the jail or prison patient, but they are in no hurry to do it. They may even make a comment that the person can just wait and, "I don't care if they hurt." I have seen nurses refuse to take care of these patients, and make a disgusted face when assigned. I have seen nurses discussing the patient and say hurtful or ugly things, or making fun of them, or saying something like

"I don't even want to know what they did, that would just make me hate them more."

Show kindness and genuine concern about their well-being. Who knows... maybe your kindness during that hospitalization will be inspirational to them and help them focus on rehabilitation. They may live in a hellish environment. Maybe your kindness will remind them of the good that is out in the world, and give them a reprieve from a hate-filled world. If you really really really want to have a heart of gold, consider that, as they live in a hellish environment, this is the closest thing to comfort, love, compassion, cleanliness, and peace they may ever see. Make their stay pleasant. You might be making a difference in somebody's life that will have far-reaching positive effects. Maybe they go back to the prison and tell the others about the amazing nurse that took care of them, and they are inspired to help others, so they start a prison ministry, or a support group for people with addiction.

Or, maybe everyone is short and rude to them in the hospital, and they decide there is no good out in the world anyway, so why even try. In nursing, you can change the world, one patient at a time. And that is no different when dealing with a prisoner. Perhaps you are even more powerful in making a positive change when dealing with these people. You never know how the smallest and most insignificant detail in your encounter may bring peace and hope to someone who desperately needs it.

Many people go to prison, and it changes many lives, both for the better and for the worse. Those who genuinely focus on rehabilitation will come back into the world and many will do good things. They are not monsters. It is not your place to judge. You are a nurse, and you will provide loving care to everyone equally.

# Chapter 11:  Pee, Poop, and Puke!!

### Cleaning the patient

I spoke in earlier chapters about the graphic nature of this book, and the graphic nature of the nurse's real-life work environment.  Well, this is where it begins.  So buckle in.

Please don't let this scare you off from a rewarding career in nursing.  My intention here is not to frighten you, but to help you prepare for what is to come.  Please don't quit nursing school because of me!!  I believe all people are capable of handling these things.  Some may struggle more than others, but everyone can eventually get used to it.  I worried a great deal about it myself, but it really wasn't a big deal after the first day.  And towards the end of my career, it absolutely had no effect on me.  I could clean up a catastrophic mess in a room, and then go eat a bowl of chili without a second thought.

The three "big P's," pee, poop, and puke... along with blood, puss, drainage, spit, snot, and farts can be your worst enemy, or in medical terms, your best friend.

It is important to desensitize to these things early.  If you work in a hospital or nursing home or home health, or really any other direct patient care setting (including specialty areas), you will be encountering some combination of these daily.

But, perhaps no other aspect of the human body plays a grander role in medical diagnostics, and continued nursing care and treatment.  There are limitless possibilities in what can be learned from the various body functions and fluids, along with the related sights and smells.

I clearly remember, when I was first considering leaving my job and applying to nursing school (and getting a job as a CNA), the fear and concern I had about this aspect of

147

the work (along with bathing patients and other similar activities). I had at least enough working knowledge from my EMT and firefighting work, along with information from friends who were in medicine, to know that this would be an obstacle to face. I remember wondering if I could do it. I remember wondering if I could ever get used to it. Well, obviously, the short answer is that yes, I could do it and I did get used to it. And I got used to it really fast.

I assume that you may be asking yourself the same questions. Or, perhaps you have already had enough experience that this is no problem for you. Either way, there is something to be learned here, so stay tuned.

I hate to use cliches, but "it is what it is." It's something that every human being on this planet has dealt with their whole lives. They just might not have dealt with it when it involves another person. There is nothing that your patients have or do (in most cases) that you don't have or do yourself. It is important to remove from your mind the image that nude bodies and their fluids are something new and different, as if you are venturing into uncharted territory, or discovering some new aspect of biology which had previously been unknown to you. You know what this is.

When I listed the words "poop, pee, and puke," I didn't have to define a single one of them. You're already well-acquainted, and have been your whole life. I have had friends who, while I was discussing something nursing related, would suddenly act surprised and shocked when I talked about this aspect of health care. It was as if they had never considered how an unconscious person is relieved of the calls of nature. As if perhaps they assumed that a comatose patient hooked to life support machinery magically got up to take a dump in the bathroom without help. Or, those particular body functions just don't happen while people are unconscious. I always had a good laugh during these enlightening conversations. The truth is, an unconscious patient pretty much craps the bed constantly.

I get a kick out of movies and shows where a person is seen waking up in a hospital room, having been there a long time, and the building is abandoned. One good example is the show "The Walking Dead." To refresh, it starts with a sheriff having been shot in the line of duty. He is in a coma of some sort in a hospital. He wakes up after many days of unconsciousness to find the hospital empty, trashed, and full of bodies. He walks outside and sees that society has collapsed, and the zombies have taken over. He was unconscious for a period of days, barricaded in a room alone, without medical care.

So, that's all fine. But, let's return to that part where he woke up after days of being comatose and receiving no medical care. First, he sure looked healthy. He didn't look critically dehydrated, as if he had been laying there for days without fluids. But, more important than the inaccurate medical nuances, is the fact that he woke up in a clean bed. If he had really been laying there for days, there would be so many layers of poop and pee in that bed, he would have needed a shovel to dig his way out.

If you have changed a baby's diaper, an adult diaper full of poop and pee is just the same, except scaled up several orders of magnitude. It requires a different technique to make the change, but it is ultimately the same thing. You, in CNA training or nursing school, will learn how to do this (if you have not already experienced it). It's very simple. It mostly involves the patient rolling (with or without assistance) side to side on the bed, while things are cleaned and changed out underneath them.

So, hypothetically, you have a patient who is laying flat in the bed. Upon entering the room, the overwhelming aroma of dookie welcomes you. So, you check, and sure enough, poop... everywhere. So, you get new sheets, absorbent pads, clean brief, towels, wet bath wipes and/or a tub of wet wash rags, or whatever supplies your facility uses, and you go to work. If it has spread up through the legs, you may start with cleaning the penis off, and/or the upper area of the vagina. This is important and will be discussed further. The first little while may be spent just soaking up and scooping out liquid stool from around the patient or between the legs. Or, the first few times the patient is rolled back and forth, the patient is not cleaned at all, and the masses of waste products are being rolled out in the soiled sheets.

You will, at some point, roll the patient onto their side, while the head of the bed is flat. You will clean their butt, and clean it well. For the immobilized patient, moisture and especially stool will break the skin down causing wounds. This is especially problematic around the anus. That skin is very sensitive to breaking down, and often times a patient who just kind of continuously "oozes" will become very raw, like a diaper rash times a hundred. But this epic diaper rash will develop into tissue death, and the eventual formation of a deep gaping wound that will not heal. If you do not know what this looks like, do an internet search for pictures of "perineal non-healing wound." (Really, you should do this search anyway, just to see it. It might be your first step in being desensitized to open wounds!)

You will have to spread butt cheeks and wipe repeatedly until everything is clean. Sometimes this process takes longer, because as soon as you roll the patient on their side and start wiping, they start pooping again. You may need to hold a rag over their backside in case they "spray" a little. Once they are finished, you continue to clean. You may toss soiled wash rags into a nearby soiled-linen container, or set them on the bed to be rolled up in the soiled sheets. Or, if using disposable wipes, you will toss these in the nearby medical waste container.

If a patient is more on the constipated side, a digital disimpaction may be needed. Now, I just used the word "digital," and so you are excited to think a computer might do this part. "Digital" actually just means you are going to use your fingers and some lubricant to help dig hardened stool out. This also may be accompanied by an enema of some sort. Some enemas are just a single bottle with a lubricated tip. The tip is pushed in, the bottle squeezed until empty, and it's done. Other enemas may require a bag of soapy water hung from an IV pole, and a tube from the bag is placed into the rectum, allowing for the water to flow in. Either way, what goes in, must come out. So you will want to have plenty of supplies ready to clean the mess. These processes are generally done with the patient lying on his or her side. If the hardened stool does not come out, you may have to lube up and stick your finger, knuckle deep, into their butt and manually manipulate the hard stool to break it down and/or pull it out.

Once the backside is pretty well clean, and ensuring the anal region is spotless, the linens under the patient will be rolled up and tucked under the patient. More towels may have to be included if the mess is pretty extensive so it doesn't go everywhere while rolling. A new set of linens will be placed on the uncovered side of the bed closest to you, and will be rolled out toward the patient. Then, the patient will be rolled over onto their other side. The soiled linens will be pulled out completely, and the clean linens can be pulled out from under the patient and wrapped over the other side of the mattress.

This process may take multiple rolls each direction to clean everything if the mess is extra large, and especially if it's mostly liquid. Use of a bedpan is similar. The patient is rolled onto their side, the pan wedged under their butt, and you roll them back onto it. Once they are finished, you roll them over to remove the pan and clean the patient. And, maybe I'm just bad at it. But it was extremely rare that I had someone use a bedpan and there was not still something that ended up on the sheets underneath them. Sometimes it's almost easier to just skip the whole bedpan thing and just make it all happen in the bed.

All of the cleaning and bathing procedures are naturally more challenging on a larger patient who is not only heavier, but has thick and deep rolls of extra flesh. This may require extra hands to just hold the legs apart, hold the rear end open, or to just help with the rolling process. Doing this on a 600 pound patient can prove extremely difficult, and may require the assistance of six nurses/CNA's, and maybe a mechanical lift. I've done this many times.

As I have said before, do not worry too much about the technical details here. You will get plenty of exposure and practice.

**Urine**

Urine contains some portion of the metabolic byproducts, or waste, that the body needs to remove. It also contains a volume of water which is pulled from the blood stream. When you study anatomy and physiology, you will find the kidneys are not actually connected to the digestive tract. So, liquids you drink do not go straight into the kidneys from the stomach for processing. The kidneys actual pull waste and fluid directly from the blood stream that is flowing through the renal circulatory system.

Amazingly, simply measuring the volume of urine output can tell us a great deal about the patient's cardiovascular status in an acute setting. With each stroke of the heart, 25% of the blood it pushes out goes into the kidneys. Those two little tiny organs get a massively disproportionate volume of the blood ejected by the heart as compared to the rest of the body. A reduction in blood flow to the kidneys, such as in dehydration and/or the body "shutting the kidneys down" (shock) in order to preserve circulating blood volume, urine production and output will be reduced or even stopped. Patients in all settings will have their urine output monitored and possibly managed. Patients in the ICU will have their urine measured hourly, or even more often. In the case that accurate hour-to-hour urine measurements are needed, a catheter may be inserted so the nurse can monitor in real-time the amount of urine coming out of the kidneys. A sudden change in urine output can alert the nurse to a developing problem requiring more assessment, testing, and possibly notification of a physician.

But, if less urine is coming out, it could be secondary to either retention or suppression. Retention means the kidneys are making urine, but there is a structural anomaly somewhere in the plumbing between the kidneys and the urethral meatus (pee hole) that is blocking the flow. Suppression means the kidneys are not making urine. So, each are problems. But the nature of those problems is very different and each points to different underlying etiologies. And, we always have to consider that there are two kidneys. So, one kidney might be suppressed while the other is not, or one may be blocked while the other is not. Sometimes a nephrostomy tube is placed, which is a catheter surgically inserted through the back and into the kidney. A patient may have one on each side. That way, urine drains directly from the kidney into an external bag, instead of hitting the blockage. And/or we may see the individual urine outputs of each kidney.

Numerous tests can be performed on urine. The concentration is measured (basically comparing the amount of dissolved "stuff" to the amount of liquid present). Very concentrated dark urine might indicate dehydration. Very thin clear urine might represent proper hydration and/or heavy diuresis (whether intended or not). Examination by the naked senses can note color, clarity, presence of sediment, presence of gross blood, and odor.

Microscopic tests can show whether there are certain

products in the urine that would indicate infection or kidney injury or other organ-specific problem, or the presence of trace blood.   White blood cells, leukocyte esterase, and nitrites can point to infection.  Protein levels in the blood can indicate an assortment of potential problems in the body. Sometimes an injury to the body can result in kidney failure because a large quantity of harmful compounds are released into the blood stream, and they overwhelm the kidneys' ability to work as a filter.

Ultimately, urine is sort of like blood, in that it is a fluid produced by, and inside, the body, and so its components and its nature can be tested in all sorts of ways for diagnostic purposes.  And in that same spirit, since it is a product of filtering and waste management, it can give clear information about metabolic processes in the body.

I have seen bright blue urine, as a result of a specific medication.  I have seen dark tea-colored or black urine, as a result of kidney damage.   I have seen a person basically urinating out pure blood.  Some people who are on dialysis produce no urine at all.  The kidneys do not function.  The dialysis procedure filters the blood and removes metabolic wastes and extra water. There are many possibilities.

Diuresis refers to the process of the body producing a larger-than-normal amount of urine.  It is often done with medications, when the body is retaining too much fluid, and thereby strain is placed on the circulatory system.  It can also be an undesired result of an acute or chronic disease process.

## Urinary Tract Infections, Perineal Care, Urinary Catheters

Women, especially if incontinent of stool, are at an increased risk for urinary tract infections versus men.  The simple fact is that the urethral meatus (opening where the urine comes out) on a woman is in the vaginal region, and can be difficult to locate.  A man's urethral meatus is on the end of the penis, so it is easier to keep clean and avoid contamination by stool.

An incontinent woman will often have stool squeezed up between her legs. This means that appropriate perineal care requires the legs to be spread, and the vagina to be spread open in order to genuinely clean all stool out of the folds and off of the urethral meatus. Stool entering the urethra can easily cause infection. It is always important to clean from front to back, so in a wiping motion, you would wipe the vagina first and then down towards the anus. If you wipe the other direction, anus to vagina, you are more likely to drag stool and germs up into the vaginal and urethral openings. Most women already know this from their own care. It remains important with men as well to clean the urethral opening, especially if stool is present. But, simple understanding of anatomy shows how the risk is higher with women for infection.

Clearly, the process of perineal care, especially on women, is an invasive procedure, and requires a great deal of personal exposure. Women may be uncomfortable with this and will have concerns about modesty, privacy, and dignity. A male nurse or CNA performing this function can add a layer of discomfort. Older females who are chronically incontinent may have no problems at all being cleaned like this. A younger female, who hasn't had this done before, will likely struggle a great deal with the process, and may refuse to let a man help. It is perfectly okay to honor a female's request for no men to be present.

However, it is done by men all the time. Some women may request a female nurse, but most others who have had to be assisted with cleaning before have desensitized to the process and are comfortable with a man doing the task. It's important for male staff to be aware of the potential for claims or accusations to be made by patients, whether they are true or not.

Brett Craigsly

I find that it is usually best, if you are a man cleaning or bathing a female of any age, to have a "chaperone," either another nurse or the CNA present to assist. When you document the procedure, you will list that person's name as being present during the process as chaperone. I have seen confused or disoriented patients say all sorts of crazy things about being attacked or otherwise physically violated. I have never had this problem cause any trouble for me, but I was always careful to have a chaperone, and so you should consider that best practice.

I will make a quick side not here. Confused patients very commonly say things that are not true, but that they believe to be true. Some are obvious, like that the nurse is an alien and the hospital is a spaceship. Others might believe they are actually in their home and you are a visitor. Or, more darkly, they may say they have been shot, beaten, raped, arrested, etc. They will hallucinate or have delusions, speak to people who are not there, and make every sort of claim imaginable.

Funny story, I was working in the ER one night and we were taking care of an overdose patient. She was awake but very confused and lashing out. There were like six of us around the bed. She suddenly pointed at me and said, "His penis is out and he's shaking it at me!" I am happy to inform you that my penis was not actually out, nor was there any recreational shaking. What was funny was the other five people (nurses and physicians) looked at me, and then looked down at my waist, as if they were checking, just to be sure. I threw my hands up and was like, "come on guys! Really?!?"

This was a funny scenario. But I had plenty of witnesses, so no worries. Now, everyone understands the nature of dealing with the confused patient. And we all know to not believe the things they say. But, it's still never good to be caught in a situation where something like that is said, and you have no witness or chaperone. I wrote an extensive nurses note in the chart describing the incident, and naming each person who was in the room.

In an unrelated situation, we had a semi-confused patient in the ICU claim that the nurse took her pain pill instead of giving it to the patient (took the pill in the patient room, right in front of the patient). We all know this is highly unlikely. However, we are required to report that sort of thing up the chain since it is an accusation involving a drug. I had to tell the hospital supervisor, and we had to pull the nurse off the floor and give her patients to someone else. A urine sample was immediately collected and sent to the lab for a drug screen. A security guard came to the unit and searched her purse and locker. I stayed with her through all of it to show support, as I totally believed she was innocent. But, I still had to send her home, and she was taken off the schedule for the next couple of shifts pending the results of her drug screening, and so the unit director, pharmacist, security officer, and risk management person could conduct their own little investigation. The drug screen was clear and the investigation deemed her innocent. There was no surprise that she was innocent. I trusted this nurse as much as any other nurse I had ever worked with. She returned to work a couple of days later. But, this goes to show how one confused patient saying one stupid (untrue) thing can create a disaster for the nurse. It's always best to protect yourself with a chaperone in a situation where something sexual could be stated. But you can't really do that with passing medications. So you just have to do your best.

In the nursing home, I saw CNA's fired a couple of times over a patient complaint, of which I questioned the validity. It was stuff like, "she hit me." I knew the CNA, and I seriously doubt she took a swing at a little old lady. But it's like the organization would rather fire the CNA and make a show of responding to the complaint, instead of taking the chance that the complaint was legitimate and they did nothing. Fire first, then do the investigation. Just always be aware of your surroundings, what patients are saying, how things look, and do your best to always protect yourself. This may mean frequently documenting the crazy things a patient says, especially if the statements involve any sort of accusation.

Okay, back to the original subject. Providing perineal care for a man can result in all sorts of other interesting scenarios. While it is not terribly common, you should be aware that a male patient may develop an erection during care, or may even begin masturbating. Whether you take this as a compliment about your looks is up to you. However, and erection is usually just an innocent biological reaction to physical stimulation, and the masturbation usually involves some sort of other mental disability that inhibits his social discretion.

A male of sound mind, who is young and healthy, might develop an erection from being touched, and they will not be able to stop it. It does not matter if they are mentally attracted to the nurse, or if they are having an unclean thought, or if they are otherwise "in the mood for love." The basic physical touch causes the erectile process to begin, even if they are trying to stop it, especially if they are younger, like teenager age range. They will likely apologize profusely. Please know that if they say they can't help it, it's because they really can't help it. Teenage males going through puberty can get erections constantly for no apparent reason. The body is suddenly ready for sex during puberty, so it likes to pop an erection as often as possible, even in the absence of sexual stimulation. An attractive girl walks by, bam...erection. The wind blows slightly, bam...erection. A car drives by, bam...erection. A documentary is on television about math, bam...erection.

If the patient confused or disabled mentally, a male patient may react sexually to the simple physical stimulation and touching, resulting in the aforementioned erection, or other acting-our behaviors such as attempting to touch or grab the female nurse inappropriately. They may also simply verbalize or otherwise physically express that they are enjoying being touched. I remember one patient in particular who, due to mental disability and social incompetence, would frequently request the female nurses to come in and hold his penis while he urinated, or clean him regularly, etc. In this particular case, the patient was perfectly capable of performing these tasks for himself, so the nurses would assist him with the setup, but then direct him to do the cleaning or holding himself.

These scenarios are usually very quickly identified as a problem, and so this is a good opportunity to have one or more additional staff members present. A male nurse or CNA may be especially useful. Whatever the case, you will always need to be aware that anything can happen, no matter how crazy or unlikely you think it might be. You can work around an erection if necessary, or ask the patient to do that cleaning for himself if he can.

If a patient becomes sexually aggressive or performs outward sexual behavior, you may leave the room and get help (assuming the patient is left in a safe manner, and will not fall or otherwise hurt themselves in your absence). Ultimately, your safety (female nurses in particular) is of highest priority, and you do not have to be subjected to sexual activities or aggression from patients. Do not let a patient touch your boobies or grab your butt. You have the right to be protected from sexual advances. These are the times you will be thankful for your male coworkers.

**Urinary Catheters**

The urinary catheter is a tube which is inserted into the urethral meatus, up through the urethra, and into the bladder. The other end of the tube attaches to a plastic bag.

The tip of the catheter in the bladder will have a small balloon inflated with sterile water or saline, which keep the tube from slipping out. Catheters have received a lot of blame in recent years as a major source of urinary tract infection, so they require constant care. Insertion of a catheter is a sterile process. You will learn how to do it in school. But, breaking sterile technique during insertion, or failing to provide proper cleaning and care, will result in infection.

A catheter may also be placed in the bladder through a surgical opening in the lower abdomen. Tubes may also be surgically inserted directly into the kidneys or ureters to bypass the bladder completely, as was mentioned earlier.

Inserting a catheter into a female is very difficult because the urethral meatus can be hard to find, and there is surrounding tissue that has to be held back out of the way. Sometimes, especially on a larger patient, you have to really get all up in there and spread things way open to find the target. Once the catheter is in the urethra, it usually goes in easily for females. But it is not safe to go in blind, and hope to hit the right spot. It is important to be able to visualize the urethral meatus and know you are inserting the catheter into the right place. If it goes into the vagina as you are repeatedly pulling and pushing, trying to hit the target, it will pick up germs that can cause infection. For males, locating the urethral opening is easy (on the tip of the penis), which also makes sterile technique easier, but threading the catheter fully into the bladder can be challenging if the patient has an enlarged prostate. Special catheters are sometimes required, and in a few cases, a urologist has to place the catheter.

A patient who has had one of several possible procedures, such as a TURP (transurethral resection of the prostate), a thicker catheter may be inserted, containing multiple inner tubing chambers, so one tube is flowing saline in to continuously irrigate the inside of the bladder, while the other tube is continuously letting the saline, urine, and blood flow out into a bag.

Like perineal care, urinary catheter insertion can be complicated in the larger patients. A large female patient may require more staff members to just hold the legs open, and hold back all of the extra flesh that surrounds the lower abdomen and vagina. Another staff member may have to hold the vagina open so the nurse with sterile gloves does not have to touch anything but the sterile catheter and equipment. On a larger man, the penis may be sort of lost inside of deep skin folds, and those folds will have to be held back. Once the folds are held back, the penis may still remain so deep in the anatomy that no actual outward penis structure is left, and the urethral opening is located deep in the tissue somewhere.

**Stool**

One might assume that the nature of poop is relatively steady. But, this is not true, and a lot can be learned by it. Hard solid stools, bulky stools, frothy stools, liquid stools, red stools, gray stools, black stools, stools with chunks of things, and stools with any one of many possible smells... These can all tell us things about the function of the digestive tract, along with other possible disease processes in the body.

One of the most common "poop problems" I saw in the ICU was the gastrointestinal bleed. A GI bleed refers to any circumstance in which bleeding (inside the digestive tract) is occurring anywhere between the esophagus down to the anal opening. And then the patient passes the blood via the anus, either with or without the presence of stool. A reasonable thought is that the brighter red blood is coming from somewhere closer to the anus, and the tarry darker black stuff is coming from somewhere up higher. Basically, blood coming from up high, like the stomach or esophagus, must traverse the entirety of the digestive tract, so what you get at the very end is a black tarry liquid substance that is a mixture of partially-digested blood and stool.  The smell of this is unmistakable, and once you experience it for the first time, you will likely always be able to identify a GI bleed just based on that magical aroma.  In fact, when going in for my shift, as soon as I stepped into the ICU hallway, I could tell you whether we had a GI bleed on the unit or not.  The smell will finds its way down the hall and around the corners. Bright red blood has not had time to mix with stool, or be digested, and so it usually is coming from the lower area, perhaps even just hemorrhoids.

If a GI bleed is up high, in the esophagus or stomach, the patient's stomach may not like its presence and decide to purge itself.  So, the patient begins vomiting blood.  If there is any concern for airway compromise, like the patient has a reduced level of consciousness, or already has problems with airway protection, they may need to be intubated and/or have a nasogastric or orogastric tube placed.  Nurses put in these tubes.  They run either up the nose or directly into the mouth, and are threaded down the esophagus into the stomach.  They are hooked to suction, so they are continuously removing all blood and keep the stomach empty.

It is important to know that a GI bleed is serious, and patients can (and do) bleed to death on occasion.  If something really opens up in there and is flowing blood, it can be difficult to get to it with a scope to stop the bleeding. And it can be difficult to stay ahead of the blood loss.  We very often give blood transfusions to patients with a GI bleed. And sometimes we give them in multiples, and fast.  We will also perform coagulation studies to check the measurable rates of blood clotting.  And we may infuse other blood products, like fresh frozen plasma or platelets to introduce more clotting factors into the blood stream.

Most GI bleeds are non-traumatic in nature.  This means that they result from an ulceration of some sort that starts to bleed.  "Stomach ulcers" are a relatively common phenomenon that most people have heard of. People tend to take an antacid for these. But if one really opens up and bleeds, it can go fast. Medical problems like portal hypertension secondary to hepatic failure can cause esophogeal varices, which are ulcerations in the esophagus. These tend to bleed very heavily. Medications, such as anticoagulants and non-steroidal anti-inflammatory drugs (aspirin, ibuprofen) can lead to bleeding.

Some cases are trauma related. I had a gun-shot case in the emergency department where man had been shot in the abdomen. The bullet had clearly pierced some part of this intestines, as he was profusely pouring blood out of his anus. He also had blood going inside his abdominal cavity. Needless to say, this patient goes straight to surgery.

Prior to GI studies, such a colonoscopy, patients are required to do a "bowel prep." This usually includes some combination of ultra high-dose osmotic or saline laxatives, oral stimulant laxatives, and/or enemas. The purpose is to have the patient passing stool so much, for so long, that they eventually are passing nothing but clear water. Then the large intestine is nice and clean for the gastroenterologist to be able to run the scope up there and have a look around. A bowel prep may be quite easy for an ambulatory patient who can constantly get up to the bathroom or just sit on a bedside commode, continuously filling it up.

But consider the immobilized patient... the patient who is unable to stand, and is bed-bound. Consider an immobilized patient that weighs 400 pounds. These are epic situations to deal with. They will just continuously pass liquid stool into the bed, for hours... like... a lot of hours. As soon as they, and the bed, are cleaned, they just keep passing stool. So it just becomes a routine that every 30 minutes to one hour they have to be bathed and have the bed linens changed, and the actual bed wiped down with disinfectant wipes. Meanwhile they just keep going. If you are not careful, it will fill up all the space under and around them and the liquid stool will start running down under their feet, and may run off the bed onto the floor. And you take care of all of this with them still in the bed.

Infectious stool is also a common presence. Many stool infections, such as clostridium difficile (C-diff), are antibiotic resistant, highly contagious, and very difficult to get rid of. They cause varying degrees of diarrhea, often have unique odors (none of which are good), and require extra isolation precautions for the patient. This means each person entering the room may have to wear a plastic gown and gloves, and maybe a mask and face shield if any "splashing" or "spraying" is expected during a cleanup. One interesting example of the hearty nature of C-diff is that its spores can live for weeks on a hard dry surface, ready to infect whoever comes in physical contact. So entire rooms are scrubbed with bleach, which is basically the only thing that can kill the spores.

In the way of infectious stool, some instances are called "opportunistic infections." The digestive tract is full of bacteria. It's mostly healthy bacteria that help digest food and have a symbiotic relationship with your body. However, a patient may have been receiving antibiotics for a long time for another infection, pneumonia for example. But the antibiotics also kill bacteria elsewhere in the body. So, the long-term use of the antibiotic kills off the healthy bacteria in the digestive tract. In its absence, other unhealthy bacteria (which are not affected by the antibiotic) have a chance to grow and thrive. C-diff is a major one like this.

I have never had experience with it, but there has emerged a medical treatment for this specific circumstance. It's called bacteriotherapy and is basically a transplant of healthy bacteria from one person into the digestive tract of the affected individual. How is that done, you ask? Well, I'll tell you. Poop transplant. We'll take poop from one person and put it in another person. Simple! Poop transplants are no longer just a fun activity on the weekends. They actually have medical value too!

This is most commonly done by colonoscopy where the gastroenterologist is able to place the stool directly into the large intestine. A less common way is by nasoduodenal tube. This is a tube inserted into the nose, run down the esophagus, and pushed through the stomach into the first portion of the small intestine. The stool transplant can then be deployed there.

Gray-colored stools don't have bile present, which gives the stool its usual pleasant brown color. This is a direct result of liver failure, as the liver is what produces the bile, or a blockage in a bile duct, so the bile does not flow into the intestine.

Nurses will frequently harvest stool samples from patient beds or bedside toilets, to be sent for testing. The presence of blood can be confirmed, along with testing for the presence of infections and parasites.

Some patients may have an "ostomy." This is a term relating to a surgical opening in the abdomen, where a bag or tube is attached to drain the contents of the intestine. A "colostomy" bag is attached to the lower intestine, and so actual stool comes out into the bag, instead of passing through the anus. Other similar surgical openings between the outer abdomen and the digestive tract are the duodenostomy, ileostomy, and the jejunostomy. Each connects to a different part of the intestine, and therefore if something is drained, it will vary depending on how much digestion has occurred. In the duodenostomy or jejunostomy, the patient may even have a feeding tube in place to provide feedings while bypassing the stomach. Colostomies and ileostomies are probably the most common you will see for the purpose of draining stool. A colostomy will produce stool, pretty much just as it would be if passed from the anus.

An ileostomy will often produce a more liquid pre-stool type substance. The bags must regularly be taken off of the patient, the ostomy site cleaned, and a new bag applied. This can be challenging if the anatomy does not allow for a clean level seal to be created. They can leak a lot.

A rectal tube is similar to a urinary catheter, except it is a larger tube that is inserted through the anus and secured in the rectum. It drains liquid stool in the case a patient has severe wounds or skin breakdown and has the continuous presence of liquid stool complicating these matters.

A patient may have a bowel obstruction, where some portion of their intestine is clogged. In these cases, the patient is not allowed to eat or drink anything, as we wait for the obstruction to clear on its own. In extreme cases, it may require surgery to fix. These patients often have a nasogastric tube in place to continuously suction the contents of the stomach so nothing is allowed to build up behind the obstruction.

Varying amounts, sizes, textures, and even shapes of stool can be useful diagnostically. Structural problems, post-surgical problems, or problems with motility can lead to constipation and/or a bowel impaction. A blockage in the digestive tract can be extremely dangerous, and if not treated correctly, lethal.

After a surgery, a patient must be monitored closely to ensure they are passing stool, or at least passing gas, so we know the digestive tract has not stopped working because of anesthesia. Post-operative constipation is common, and bowel obstructions are a risk, if certain precautions are not taken.

When choosing between constipation and diarrhea, we always choose diarrhea. As long as the patient is kept hydrated (even by IV fluids) and their electrolyte balances are kept appropriate, diarrhea is completely tolerable. However, constipation can be extremely dangerous. It can quickly and easily evolve into a legit bowel obstruction, which is quite serious. People can die from bowel obstructions and impactions. So, it is very rare that you will see any medications given in the hospital that would stop diarrhea, such as Immodium. But there are tons of medications that will cause diarrhea, and you will give those often.

A couple of examples are lactulose and kayexalate. If a patient is in acute or chronic liver failure, they will have an unsafe buildup of ammonia in their blood stream. This is easily detectable with simple blood tests. It generally comes with high levels of confusion and disorientation. So, any time you have a chronic liver patient start to act confused, an ammonia level is usually one of the first things we check (of course, don't worry about this, the physician makes the decisions and writes the orders). The lactulose causes epic diarrhea, which flushes the ammonia out via the stool. Lactulose is often dosed based on the number of liquid bowel movements it produces in a day.

Kayexalate binds with potassium in the digestive tract, pulling it out of the blood, and excreting it in stool (also in the form of epic diarrhea). So, among many other treatments, it is a very common drug used in a patient with dangerously high potassium levels.

**Vomit**

This was always the hardest one for me. I could deal with it, but it never got quite as easy as the others. As referenced earlier, a person may vomit blood, instead of it going the other way. Vomit may be collected and tested for the presence of blood. It can sometimes be difficult to determine if red vomit is blood or just spaghetti sauce from lunch. Frequent vomiting can be extremely dangerous in some cases. An unconscious or sedated patient, or patient with existing swallowing problems can very easily choke on vomit. It actually happens frequently. Many pneumonia cases that come into the hospital are immobilized or unconscious patients, or those who are unable to swallow and/or have a feeding tube. They have essentially vomited and choked on it. The amount that got into the lungs has now caused "aspiration pneumonia" which can be quite dangerous.

Patients who are deeply sedated and on a ventilator, will often have an orogastric or nasogastric tube inserted through the mouth or nose, threaded down the esophagus, and the tip is positioned in the stomach. It can then be connected to suction to continuously evacuate the stomach of blood or gastric juices, in order to prevent vomiting and protect the airway. Or it can essentially keep the digestive tract completely empty for other GI-related problems, like obstructions or surgeries.

You may have to consider things like whether a patient vomited up the pills you just administered moments before. Perhaps you will need to dig through the vomit to try and locate the pills. If they are found and clearly identified, you may need to give them again (new pills obviously).

**Blood and the rest**

Blood is pretty obvious here. We all know that constant blood tests are a fixture in healthcare, and in a higher-acuity environment testing may happen continuously. Drawing blood may be done by a nurse, a specially trained CNA, or a phlebotomist. It just depends on your facility's staffing structure on who does the job.

Many patients may have a post-operative drain placed. This might be a tube running into a specific place in the abdomen, for the purpose of continuously draining blood or puss, etc. It has to be examined and measured frequently, and the tube often has to be flushed with saline.

Another major example is the chest tube. A chest

tube goes though the chest wall and into the space between the lungs and chest wall. It is hooked to suction and continuously drains air, blood, puss, etc. This is a primary treatment for a collapsed lung, and is also used in open-chest surgeries. A mediastinal tube is the same thing, but it goes into the area around the heart.

Every other sort of liquid, juice, discharge, drainage, mass, growth, or surgically-removed structure in the body can be tested in many ways.

As always, please remember that this is not meant to be used as a reference in your future decision making or practice as a nurse. There are usually multiple variables that can cause any problem. So, don't let my examples here guide you. In your practice, you should rely on the formal education you receive in school, your hospital policies and protocols, your own knowledge and experience, your nursing intuition, and the orders received from physicians.

# Chapter 12:   Specialists and Audits

I must give my usual disclaimer here.  I have been out of the game for a couple of years, and so it's always possible that things have changed within boards of nursing, state regulations and laws, and oversight/certifying agencies. Also, I just have my limited experience with my hospital system and a couple of other employers.  I can't guarantee that all of this is still accurate, small details may vary between employers, and regulations may vary among different states, and so you would need to check with your hospital policies and procedures.

I realize that this is perhaps the most boring of the discussions to be had in this book.  But this is important stuff. You don't need to fully grasp all of these concepts to start your nursing career.  The one thing to really take away from this chapter is the information about compliance and "best practice" standards.  So please pay special attention there. Those are things that will directly affect you the first day you start working as a nurse.

I talked earlier about "case-specific specialists" and how they relate to hospital business and the various government and oversight agencies.

Hospitals and other healthcare facilities are not just independently operated however the management sees fit, and the physicians do not work however they want, and the nurses don't just blindly do what the hospital and physicians instruct.   Like many other trades, those who work in healthcare generally will be licensed in some way, from the CNA certification up to the medical license of the Chief Medical Officer.   In fact, the vast majority of positions require some sort of license or certification to do the job. This means that each different type of employee may have to report to a different certifying board or agency, and the work they do will have to fit correctly with the work everyone else does. Further, there are standards set in the medical community, nation and world-wide.

So, a hospital will have hands from many different outside agencies and states reaching in to control those aspects in which they are involved. They might be specific to a single position, or a facility, or a whole system. Hospitals, and their staff, must work in tune with all of these outside agencies and government entities, which seek to set an overall standard which every system must follow. This part is boring, but hang with me.

Procedures, policies, practices, facilities management, and documentation (among many other aspects) all must meet a certain standard set by these outside organizations, with the goal being to promote the best possible care for the patient, in each existing system and facility.

Take for example a hypothetical hospital, where a patient is treated for a heart attack. The physician personally does not believe in the need for an ace inhibitor in addition to a beta blocker and/or a calcium channel blocker when discharging the patient with new prescriptions. The physician also thinks the whole thing with aspirin is no good. So, he or she writes the orders the way they want, and send the patient on their way. In another hospital, the physician includes these other medications on a similar heart attack patient (as this is the established standard for best practice). So, we have two reasonably identical patients, being treated two different ways. Will one of them have problems and not the other, or will one even die as a result of their physician's personal preferences? One of the physicians diverted from the details of treatment that have been widely accepted as the best practice. Is he smarter than everybody else? Or has he put his patient at risk by leaving the established process and having marched off in his own direction?

If a patient walks into a hospital, should they have to ask to see the policies and procedures in order to assure themselves they have patronized the right facility? Should they have to worry about knowing the "good hospital" from the "bad hospital" in town? Ultimately, the answer is no. In a perfect world, all hospitals would take care of patients the exact same way, and achieve the exact same high standard of care and positive outcomes.

Hospitals will advertise to attract more patients, however, in the case that you were having a heart attack, should you have to stop and research the best hospital in town to save your life? Again, no.

These examples show the need for the assurance of quality in all systems and facilities. If a facility is licensed and certified to be open for business, it has to meet very strict standards. These standards stretch far and deep into the inner workings of the organization.

Hospital policies and practices will include very specific rules in documentation, time spent during and between procedures, other aspects of care plans, nurse-patient education, followup appointments, medication recommendations, and re-admissions. For example, there are goals called "door to needle" or "door to cath," in which timing is monitored for each step in a series of processes in taking care of a heart attack or stroke patient. Documentation must reflect that from the time a chest pain patient physically enters the hospital, an EKG, certain blood tests, certain imaging studies, the initiation of certain medications and intervention all must occur in narrowly-defined times.

These may not currently be accurate, so don't hold me to it, but each of these is a measurement from the time the patient enters the hospital to the time a task is completed... so for "door to cath", patient physically enters the ER with chest pain. An EKG must be taken and interpreted by physician within five minutes, blood test results returned and reviewed by physician within 30 minutes, a chest x-ray performed and reviewed by a radiologist within 30 minutes, bedside consultation and exam by the interventional cardiologist within 40 minutes, and initiation of cath lab procedure within 60 minutes. There are also specific cardiac medications to be administered in there somewhere once a true serious heart attack has been diagnosed.

For a stroke patient, the "door to needle" process starts when they arrive in the hospital.... EKG completed and read by physician within five minutes, lab work interpreted by physician within 30 minutes, CT scan of the head without contrast taken and interpreted by a radiologist within 30 minutes, a neurologist consultation at bedside or via video-chat at the bedside within 40 minutes, and initiation of TPA or Alteplase (drug to dissolve blood clot in the brain) within 60 minutes.

Take the chest pain case for example, let's assume the patient was having a heart attack and his life was saved as he was in the cath lab within 60 minutes. Every step of the way, the nurse, the ER physician, the laboratory staff, the EKG technician, the radiology technicians, the radiologist, the interventional cardiologist, and the cath lab nurses must have perfect and accurate documentation, showing every single detail of every single activity at every single moment, while also reviewing and documenting all of the other assessment data, medical history, and related information that would help direct care.

Meanwhile, they are doing all of the other expected stuff, like changing the patient into a gown, hooking him up to all of the monitoring equipment, starting IV's, drawing the blood, initiating IV infusions of live-saving medications, transporting the patient between the ER and the cath lab, talking to the panicked wife, talking to the panicked patient, getting the consent paperwork signed by the patient, and ultimately each team member coordinating with each other team member for everything to be done correctly, in order, with no steps missed, and within set time limits.

So, our hypothetical patient survived his heart attack. He has now been transferred from the cath lab to the ICU. After a predetermined period of time, and after meeting certain criteria in blood tests for clotting, the ICU nurse will have to extract the introducer device that has been surgically placed in the large femoral artery of the patient's leg. This device allowed the cardiologist to thread different equipment into the artery and up into the heart. The exact procedure for this removal is critical so the patient does not bleed to death. It usually takes at least 45 minutes for the nurse to complete this delicate procedure. No physician is present. Once removed, the site of the introducer and the circulation to the leg must be evaluated and documented, along with several other components like vital signs, every 15 minutes for two hours, and then every 30 minutes for four hours, and then every hour for 12 hours, and then every four hours for 24 hours. Vital signs will also follow this schedule.

The patient must have been started on a specific set of medications, whose use has been determined to be "best practice" by the greater medical community, within some specific period of time. Certain blood tests and followup EKG's must be performed within certain periods of time. The nurse must provide (and document) certain components of education regarding the procedure, expected changes in the patient's activity level, new medications, new lifestyle changes, and other aspects of home and followup care. The nurse must have prepared certain aspects of a heart attack-related nursing care plan in the chart. The physician must document their followup teaching and patient instructions. The physician must discharge the patient on a set of specific medications, or have clearly documented the valid reasons why he or she has made changes to this normal practice.

This all happens while, somewhere in there, the

doctors and nurses are still "taking care" of patients.

So, this is just one of countless examples of "best practice" standards that have been set. Hospitals are expected to follow this procedure exactly. Once completed, the "Chest Pain/STEMI Coordinator" in the hospital will review every detail of the case, from start to finish, along with all documentation. Any problems located will be noted and they will usually follow up with the unit leadership about where they see problems. It is literally as little as a failure to write down a (perfectly normal) temperature among the vital signs at the exact right time for a certain patient. If it is written one minute too late, it's wrong. If it is written one minute too early, it's wrong. Basically, perfection is expected.

One quick note on the perfection of the charting. The computer systems allow the nurse to chart things after they happen. So, let's say you make an assessment of the introducer site, and then get busy doing something else. You later sit down and document your assessment, but change the time stamp to show the time it was done, not the time you are actually documenting it. So, if you took a temperature reading at 7:59 a.m. and it was actually due at 8:00 a.m., you had better time-stamp it for 8:00 a.m., or it's wrong. Details details details!!!

This exact example brings up a series of paradoxical frustrations in nursing. We are presented with all of these standards, protocols, procedures, rules, regulations, time lines, and practices. We are expected to chart something with the time stamp of the exact time it was due to occur. Can we claim that we did those cath site assessments every 15 minutes, on the dot, every time? No, there will always be a few minutes early or a few minutes late here and there. It's the nature of the business. You might have two or three or five other patients under your care. Do the systems and auditors really believe we did those activities at the exact right moment? I don't know.

The nursing text book will teach you that if you find your patient sitting in bed crying... do you...

A) Leave them alone to have private time

 B) Tell then everything is going to be okay

C) Sit quietly with them at the bedside and allow them to discuss their concerns

D) Call the family to come be with them

The correct answer is C. So, let's say you are sitting with your crying patient as the text book instructs. Meanwhile, your 15-minute cath site check is due. Also, another patient is pushing the call light. Also, The ER is trying to call report to send up your new patient. Also, the charge nurse is trying to get your shift report with updates on your patients. Also, you need to pee really bad and have been so busy you haven't been to the bathroom in hours.

Does the greater nursing system, the text books, the educators, the leadership, the outside auditors, the state, and oversight agencies.... do they all really believe that you are checking that cath site at exact perfect 15 minute intervals? Or does it only matter that the paperwork is perfect? I always say that when you are in nursing school, and when taking the NCLEX licensing exam, answer every question with the underlying assumption that you have unlimited time, unlimited resources, no other patients, no phone calls, no interruptions, and no other place to be. So, you can sit at the side of the bed and listen to your crying patient talk... since that is the right answer on the test.

When I was working in the nursing home, and the state inspectors were there for an annual visit, one of them approached me and wanted to watch me give medications to one of my patients. Okay, fine, no problem.

So, I washed my hands. I unlocked and opened my medication cart. I pulled up the patient's medication documentation record. I carefully pulled each medication out of its holder and placed it in the cup while checking each dose and expiration date, and re-checked each medication, expiration date, and dose twice (so three total checks). I completed the appropriate documentation on the medication administration record in the chart. I closed and locked the medication cart. I closed the medical chart.

Then, I knocked on the resident's door, which was already wide open. He looked at me like I was crazy but shrugged his shoulders and went back to his television. I announced that it was Brett, the nurse, and that I was coming in to give his scheduled medications. He looked at me like I was crazy again. I stopped at the sink and washed my hands again. I then approached the guy, and asked him to tell me his name, and I checked his wrist band (two patient identifiers). Again, he looked at me like I was crazy. I stated the names of the medications I was giving him, along with their doses. I watched him take the pills. I asked him if he had any questions or concerns about the medications. He looked at me like I was crazy. I asked him if there was anything else I could do for him. I did a quick safety check of his room and surroundings. I made sure he had the call light in reach. I returned to the sink and washed my hands. Then I exited the room.

The guy kept looking at me like I was crazy because I had given him the same medications every day for months. So, he was not used to me making a big show of introducing myself and discussing the medications with him.

It was an absolutely perfect performance on how to give medications, according to the text book. The only problem was it took like 10 or 15 minutes from start to finish. So, let's do math. I have 30 residents. Each receives medications at least twice during my shift, some even more. But, let's just say that is 60 medication administrations total I have to do. If each takes 10 minutes, then... we get 600 minutes spent passing medications. (Don't forget some are more complex and require checking vital signs and blood sugar levels, etc). But just to keep it simple, 60 times 10 minutes each is 600 minutes, which is 10 hours. My shift is only eight hours long.

And, that does not include wound care treatments, paperwork on residents coming and going for appointments, dialysis, and outings with family, etc. It does not include the paperwork and assessment done on a new resident who moves into the facility that day. It does not include the times I get called in a room to give a pain medication. It dose not include the time I have to spend in the dining hall during supper to check each patient receives the correct meal order (not the food itself, but if it is whole, chopped, pureed, if liquids are thickened, etc, for patients with swallowing problems). It does not include the time I spend cleaning and managing catheter and colostomy bags. It does not include the time I spend talking to patient families on the phone or in person. It does not include the time I spend managing tube feedings for those patients. It does not include the time I spend in the care planning meeting at the beginning of each shift. It does not include the time I spend dealing with an emergency, or a fall, or a complaint of chest pain and sending the patient to the hospital... The list goes on. If you follow me here... It seems like the math does not work. If I do everything exactly perfect per textbook instructions, it will probably take upwards of 16 or 18 hours to do all of these chores, inside my eight hour shift.

So, back to my original point. The system and state and oversight agencies are looking for perfect documentation, and I assume they are believing that reflects perfect adherence to those scheduled activities. You see the theoretical problem with all of that.

Anyway, I don't have an answer for you. But it is important that you understand this dynamic and paradox. These are the expectations. You have to get the job done.

You have to find a way. But you have to be safe. You have to take good care of your patients and you must avoid mistakes. You must wash your hands constantly, just like in my nursing home example. You must double-check everything. Being "too busy" or "short on time" is not an acceptable excuse for mistakes, mis-timed medications, or failure to adhere to basic practices like hand-washing between patients.

Please let me be very clear. I am not encouraging you to cut corners. I am not encouraging you to break rules. I am not encouraging you to do things wrong. I am telling you that you still have to do things the right way. But, be prepared for that to be a challenge a lot of the time. I worked with a nurse who used to tell me in report I "better had brought my roller skates today." The implication is that I would be running so fast to get everything done, roller skates would get me up and down the hallway faster than walking. For you younger folks, roller skating was something we old people did when we were kids before there were video games. Look it up on the internet.

Back to our heart attack patient from earlier. The chest pain/STEMI coordinator who oversees the processes you are doing will work with the nursing departments, the physicians, the individual staff, the education department, the other specialists (like quality coordinator), and upper management, while also attending all sorts of committee meetings on policies, procedures, practices, and problem resolution.

So, the patient survived and went home. Numerous members of the staff have collectively spent hours performing and documenting every imaginable detail at excruciatingly exact times. No detail was missed. The "chest pain/STEMI Coordinator" checks that one off. And... Then we repeat this process over and over, multiple times a day. This is just for one specific patient. The hospital still has hundreds of other patients with hundreds of other problems, each requiring their own "best practice" standards of care, case specialist to monitor and audit, and committees to discuss.

The "case specialists," as I have called them, each have some area they focus on, and then may work together with other similar cases or committees. The "Code Coordinator" will review every case where a "rapid response" or "code blue" is called. Again, they examine every detail of the process, audit every detail of the paperwork, follow up with anybody who wasn't perfect, and use the gathered information to further improve policies and practices via committee meetings.

I have sat on lots of committees that worked on this sort of thing. For a couple of years, I was assigned to a large committee that was mostly made up of physicians (and mostly the physicians who were leaders of their specialization for the hospital). Otherwise, the Chief Medical Officer, CEO (sometimes), and the Chief Nursing Officer were there. These meetings were all totally occupied by the high-rollers and the powerful people in the system. Then I was there too. It was intimidating. I was the only nurse, outside of the Chief Nursing Officer, and sometimes a few Directors. But, mostly just doctors, executives, and me. I was told they wanted one charge nurse on the committee to sort of represent the general patient-care nursing staff. They would discuss the really high-level hospital business here, as it pertained to patient care. All of the data gathered in audits and by specialists and financial people would all funnel up to this group, who then made big decisions. We would look at crazy statistics that I never fully understood, shifts in trends over time, individual cases where something problematic happened, etc. Most of it was over my head. I'm still not even sure why they made me go. I felt useless in there. However it was an honor to be chosen for the task.

Ultimately, all of this talk about the heart attack patient and his care, the case specialists and their activities, the audits, the investigations, the exercises in root cause analysis, the committees, and the communication that occurs between all of the departments and leadership, is all centered around providing the best possible care according to national standards.

A lot of work and financial investment clearly goes into quality control.

This all seems great, and should provide comfort to patients who are cared for in hospitals. However, it doesn't stop there. Auditors and inspectors from a variety of different oversight and government agencies visit throughout the year. And they spend great quantities of time and effort going through individual cases, the way an accounting auditor might dig through financial records to trace every penny and make sure nothing inappropriate has happened. So our documentation must be tight. It's not just for the inner workings of the hospital, but it is also relied upon to keep us certified and licensed to stay in business.

I will not name any of these oversight agencies. However, I will say that they are thorough, and create a stressful atmosphere when they are present. Hospitals often have "practice surveys" with other outside inspectors to get an idea of where they are before the real inspectors arrive. My hospital usually did pretty well. I remember one survey in the ICU, we had two dings on the record. One was because they found an opened bottle of non-sterile lubricant that did not have the date it was opened written on it. The bottle was small, about the size of standard pill prescription bottle. The other problem was that there were a couple of cardboard boxes sitting directly on the floor in one of the supply rooms instead of at least several inches above the floor on a shelf. Details details details!!!

Next, there are lower, and more specific designations

that a hospital can receive. And there is a constant battle to obtain these certifications, and then to not lose them. I have referred to the Level I Trauma Center. The Level I thing is a certification that we can receive literally anything in our emergency department. It means we have a neurosurgeon on call to do emergency brain surgery, or a cardiothoracic surgeon to do an emergency heart surgery, among many others. In my trauma center, we received burn patients, but after stabilizing them we would have to fly them out to a burn center in another city. We did not have our own burn unit.

Our hospital was designated as a "chest pain" and "stroke" receiving facility. This means that the ambulances and other hospitals knew we had a cath lab that could take care of heart attacks 24 hours a day, as well as the neurologist and neurosurgery presence to handle strokes immediately. If a chest pain patient were taken to a hospital without an active cath lab, then the patient would have to be packaged up and transferred again once the heart attack is discovered, wasting a lot of precious time. This is one of those reasons why it is better to call an ambulance than drive in an emergency. The ambulance staff can establish the suspicion of the heart attack right in your living room, and then know the right place to take you. Otherwise, you may very well show up at a hospital that can do nothing for you and your specific problem. So, again, the case specialists worked closely with these certifying agencies to obtain and maintain designations.

Finally, I will mention that some of these specialists, such as the infection control coordinator, will act as an expert reference for things related to their focus. They may provide classes or training during periods of annual skills testing, inspect the hospital for correct infection control procedures, and even inspect patients and rooms for application of those procedures. Another example might be a wound care coordinator, who would perform routine inspections of patients, as compared to their charts for accuracy in nursing documentation, and would provide expert support for all things wound or skin care. The list goes on and on. A whole book could be written just about what a few of these people do. But they are basically the people who are double-checking a lot of your work to make sure it is correct.

This is all a good example of how much work goes on behind the scenes in a hospital, and how truly complicated the system is. There are lots of nurses who do not perform direct patient care, but who remain an integral part of maintaining hospital and patient care excellence.

# Chapter 13:   Nurse-Patient Relationship

## Personal Care and Intimate Interactions

When I use the word "intimacy" in this book, I am not talking about romantic or sexual intimacy.  Intimacy in this setting is all about becoming acquainted with the aspects of a patient which are usually kept secret, covered, hidden, or otherwise private.

Many patients are vulnerable and need extensive care to cover all their needs.  I have already discussed at length the nature of bathing, cleaning poop and pee, performing bowel preps, etc.  So I will not go into further detail on that aspect.  However, beyond the physical skill or activity being performed by the nurse, you have to remember that a human being is on the receiving end of it.  They may be totally awake and ambulatory and generally live a normal life.  Or they may be an elderly long-time nursing home patient who has been incontinent for years.

This is mostly common sense.  A patient who has had their brief changed due to incontinence for years will be totally fine and does not care who does it.  But, let's say an otherwise normal and healthy teenage girl is in an accident.  Maybe she is even the prom queen or homecoming queen or whatever.  But, due to trauma sustained in a car accident, she has to remain in bed and can't get up to use the bathroom.  Can you imagine what it must be like for her to have to suddenly wear a brief or use a bedpan and pass stool and urine, essentially in the bed?

Many young females would likely not handle this well.  Would they want a 40-something male nurse like myself opening everything up and cleaning them?  Probably not.  So, it is best to have females take cases like that.  Similarly, in the labor and delivery department, you generally do not see male nurses. Part of the job in that department is to be constantly inserting fingers into the vagina to check dilation and effacement during labor. A younger female of child-bearing age usually does not like a strange old man putting his fingers all up in there.

Likewise, a young male patient may prefer a man take care of him, because he can't imagine pooping in a bedpan in front of a pretty female nurse. Nothing is ever certain, but these are the types of things to consider when working with patients in that context. And always remember to have a chaperone to protect you in case a confused patient makes wild fictitious claims.

You may have to work a little to get and uncomfortable patient to cooperate, but this is always done in a calm, patient, understanding, and respectful manner. If you become impatient, it makes things way worse.

You might calmly say, "Hey, I know this must be terribly unpleasant for you. I know it would be unpleasant for me to have it done too. But doing this is important to take care of your (fill in the blank problem). I will talk you through it, and we will get it done together. (If a male nurse is speaking to a male patient) You don't have any body parts that I don't also have. And your body doesn't do anything that my body doesn't also do. I know this is super weird for you, but I do this constantly, and I know you can do it, and I know we can get through it together..."

If family is present in the room, you may have to ask the patient if they are comfortable with the family being present, or if they prefer family members leave the room. You always make sure the door and/or curtains are closed. Protect their privacy like you would protect your own privacy. And, when possible, always drape exposed body parts with a towel. If you are doing a bed bath on a female, and they are completely nude, cover their breasts and/or pelvic regions with a towel when not directly working on that area. Try to limit exposure of body parts to only when necessary. Don't sling the door or curtains open while the patient is exposed, to ask the nurse in the hall to come help. And as always, you need the patient's permission to do anything. Explain what needs to be done, and then ask them politely if you may proceed. If they are a female and you are a male, tell them up front that a female can come do the job if they are uncomfortable. Don't let them feel trapped, like you are about to do something to them, and they have no choice. A female patient has the right to not let a male provide care to her. And we must respect that right.

## General Aspects of Providing Care

You must approach all scenarios with patience, compassion, and understanding. You can't force tasks. It may take time for the patient to get comfortable with the concept before allowing the care to proceed. This is okay. If it's not a life-threatening emergency, give them the time and space they need. Never ever ever make "sigh" noises or take a heavy breath that would suggest impatience. Do no roll your eyes or shake your head in frustration. We, as nurses, quickly desensitize to the work and interactions. We forget what it must be like to be on the other end.

Imagine you are laying in a hospital bed, having passed stool, and needing to be cleaned up. You have never had this done to you before. Imagine the nurse rushes in like he or she is in a hurry. "Okay let's do this, I'm in a hurry, come on, roll over."

When you (as the patient) hesitate or want to ask questions, the nurse sighs and he/she rolls their eyes, looks at their watch, and their mind has clearly gone somewhere else.

Imagine them saying, "Well, it's now or never. I have other stuff to do. Hurry up. It's no big deal, just spread your legs..."

It does not require much imagination to see how the

patient experience is far different from the nurse experience. We clean poop all day every day. No big deal. But, the patient does not have poop cleaned off of them all day every day. Be sensitive to their experience. They are already going through a difficult injury or illness. Do not make them feel uncomfortable, as if they are a burden and you would rather not be helping them. In reality, yes, you have like 14 other places you need to be right then. But, the worst thing you can do to a patient (other than kill them) is to hurt them emotionally. Even the slightest of eye-rolling, sighing, glancing at a watch, or tapping of a foot can make the patient feel really awful.

Similarly, when cleaning poop or bathing or doing something else gross or intimate, always maintain a professional face. If you stand over the patient, wiping foul-smelling stool, and they look up and see you have a disgusted look on their face, imagine how that makes them feel. They already feel vulnerable and scared and uncomfortable having something done to them, and now they know you think they are disgusting.

I will give a hypothetical, assembled from a couple of real scenarios I saw. A former member of the military suffered a brain injury during combat. They were hit in the head by a piece of shrapnel, but survived. They now can't walk, are confined to a bed, have lost the use of one half of their body, are incontinent, have messed up speech and a disfigured face. We know that our country owes them a debt of gratitude for their service and personal sacrifice. Then, they are laying in a hospital bed, and the nurse shows signs of impatience, or makes faces when having to clean poop.

Then, after cleaning up, the nurse is going to put a brief on the patient (adult diaper). So, the nurse says, "okay, let's roll you over so I can put your diaper on." The nurse could not express the simple courtesy of using a more adult-friendly and dignified word like "brief" instead of "diaper." I have watched (in a real scenario like this) a patient's head drop to their chest in shame, embarrassment, loss of self esteem, and realization that they are now being treated like a baby instead of a wounded combat veteran, because the nurse said "diaper" instead of "brief." I was a CNA at the time. I have never forgotten that interaction, and I have never made that mistake.

Remember that every move you make is seen by the patient and by the family. Even the slightest show of impatience, lack of concern, disgust, or disinterest can be devastating. The details make or break the whole experience for the patient and family.

## Communicating With Patients and Families

It is important to instill a sense of trust in the patient and family. You need them to trust you. And you must do a good job for them. If they don't trust you, the whole system breaks down. Would you want to leave your child or spouse or parent in the care of a nurse you did not trust? Would you be scared for their safety? Not a safety issue from being mistreated, but perhaps by just being ignored?

One practice I developed when I worked in Med/Surg, and carried it all the way up into the ICU, was to immediately communicate with my patients once shift-change report is complete. Many nurses like to sit and review records, make lists of the upcoming chores, or finish their coffee. Or, sometimes a nurse will start with their first patient, doing vital signs, assessment, documentation, medications, and treatments. Then they will move to the next patient. By the time they get to the sixth patient, maybe two hours has passed, which is concerning from the perspective of the patient and family. Plus, you have taken over the responsibility and liability of care, and allowed time to pass without even laying eyes on a patient. Many hospitals now require their nurses to go room to room and give report at the bedside, for this exact reason.

So, immediately upon finishing report, I would go room to room. I would knock, stick my head in... "Hey, I'm Brett and I will be your nurse tonight. I just wanted to check in and say hello really quickly before I get started on all my routine chores. Do you have any immediate questions or concerns I can address? No? Okay then, I will be back soon to get vitals and do an assessment and we will see what else is on the schedule for you."

This very simple act and patient interaction will build more confidence in your patient and family than any show of expert skill. I have, so many times, done this, and as I am walking away from the room, I hear a family member or the patient say, "Oh, he's nice, I like him." They don't know anything about me, certainly not enough to decide to like me. But I have given them the attention needed so they know I am going to be there for them.

In other cases, the patient may know that shift change happened, but they have not seen their new nurse yet, and it's been two hours. They begin to wonder if they were forgotten, and perhaps don't even have a nurse. Sometimes just by showing up, expressing interest in their needs, and telling them you will be back later, you have made an immense stride in building the working relationship. And it took literally 30 seconds.

Sometimes they do have a need. Perhaps they ask for pain medicine, or needed to have their brief changed. As long as it is not a life-threatening emergency, you say, "Okay, great, I will take care of that very shortly. I'll be back in a few minutes. You then finish checking on your other patients, taking another one or two minutes, and you can get back to the needs of the first patient. And after this quick introduction and "check-in," you may not show back up for two hours because you are so busy, but they know you are there and will relax more easily.

## Humor and Jokes

We become desensitized to hospital life, injury, illness, and death. We become able to walk out of a room filled with tragedy and joke around at the nurse station. We are no longer phased by the things we see.

We drink too much coffee and are in a great mood, and we walk into our patient's room and say, "hey, I'm Brett, I'll be your nurse, but it will cost you a thousand bucks. Nah, I'm kidding. I hope you will behave yourself tonight (while playfully shaking a finger at them). Bro, your blood pressure sucks, let's do something about that. Wow, it looks like a bomb went off in this room."

Then, in response to a patient question about something being wet, maybe the table or something from a spilled drink, the nurse playfully says, "yeah, it's no big deal, I like it wet..." (Obvious sexual reference here) (I have witnessed this exact one happen in my ICU. The family was so pissed! I had to take the nurse off the case.) "Oh, it smells pretty ripe in here, we better check your brief. Oh, you don't need pain medication right now? No big deal, I didn't want to give it to you anyway, Ha ha ha..."

These things are intended to be friendly and funny. But they are still inappropriate. Remember, the audience watching your stand-up comedy routine is sick, injured, or maybe dying. Maybe they were just told a half hour before that they had terminal cancer and would not leave the hospital alive. You think they care about your sense of humor?

I personally have a good sense of humor. However, I also know that if I am in a bad mood or otherwise not interested in humor, attempts by others at humor not only fail to cheer me up, but will actually piss me off even more.

Every interaction with patients should begin ultra-professional. As time goes by, and the relationship develops, you will learn the nuances of the patient.

Maybe they like all these jokes and are going to say something funny every time you walk into the room. "Oh boy, here comes the vampire again to take my blood. My shit is gross, they better pay you a lot to clean me up. Hey, you're a male nurse, you're not going to try to make out with me are you?"

Your response to all of this can be playful and soft. And you may participate a little. However, things can change immediately. Maybe the patient is bipolar and is in a manic phase, but is about to get angry or depressed, and you need to be ready to change your attitude and approach as their personality changes.

Attempts at humor by a patient might also be a psychological coping mechanism. Maybe they just got the worst news imaginable. Their mind is in such shock and horror that they say something funny as an attempt to just keep from imploding in on themselves. But if you respond by initiating your stand-up comedy routine, it will make things worse. Sometimes the best response to a funny statement is not a laugh. Instead, make eye contact to see what their face is telling you, give a polite smile and head nod. Acknowledge their joke, but do not use it as a spring board for more comedy. And in some cases, although the patient statement is said in the form of a joke, the patient really has no intention of getting a laugh from it. And perhaps not even a smile is the appropriate response.

Patient: "The doctor told me this afternoon that I have pancreatic cancer and won't leave the hospital alive. I guess I won't have to worry about those overdue library books now."

Nurse: "Hahahaha, yeah, screw the library, not your problem now. By the way, I have a funny story about library books..."

In this example, the nurse clearly handled it wrong. But even a smile or laugh would not have been an appropriate response to the patient's "joke" about the overdue library books. In this scenario, the best response by the nurse would not have been humor or smile-based at all. Perhaps eye contact with a concerned and caring face, and a nod of understanding... an acknowledgment of the pain... It was not a joke, it was an expression of deep pain and suffering thinly disguised as a joke.

You may also see nurses and CNA's playfully picking at each other or joking while in the presence of a patient. This can be just about as bad. Always assume the patient is not interested in your comedy routine. They are at the hospital for a different reason than you. They are not your coworkers, they are your customers. And they are sick, injured, and/or dying. Treat them respect and professional courtesy. And keep all interactions with your coworkers professional while in the presence of a patient. The patient deserves it.

## Miscellaneous Considerations

In the case that you and your coworkers are bilingual, do not speak in another language in front of the patient. It may be a totally casual conversation that has nothing to do with the patient, but it will always make them uncomfortable. They don't know what you are saying, and they assume it's about them.

Don't walk into patient rooms and start doing stuff without first identifying yourself. "I'm Brett, one of the other nurses here. Your nurse is tied up, so she asked me to come check on you and see if you needed more pain medication." If you are the primary nurse, and you bring other staff to help you with something, introduce them.

Knock on the door before walking in. Don't barge into rooms unless you are on your way to do CPR. Don't flip on bright overhead lights without telling the patient you are going to do it. I know this stuff all sounds like common sense, but it's all stuff that I constantly saw, even from experienced nurses in the ICU. Picture if it was your own family member lying in that bed. How would you want them treated?..... Okay, now go treat your patients the same way.

## Personal Connections and Relationships

The rules are pretty simple.

You are the nurse, they are the patient. You are not friends, you are there to work for them. Your problems don't matter. Leave your personal life in your car when you enter the hospital.

If a patient says, "wow, you look tired."

Don't say, "Yeah, had a crazy night, tons of beer." Or "My husband left me and I have been up crying all night." Or "I have a sick kid in the hospital, and so instead of sleeping last night I was in the pediatric unit down the hall and awake all night with my kid."

If you have a problem significant enough to affect your ability to do the job, you should communicate it with your charge nurse or manager or director. Don't drag your problems into a patient's room.

Similarly, a patient may show genuine interest in your life. What do you do on your days off, do you work a second job, are you married, kids, how do you like nursing, and will you go on a date with my nerdy grandson? Try to refrain going into detail.

"Yeah, I like nursing, it's hard work but been very fulfilling." "I do a little work on the side in home health or on another unit." "Yeah, married and everything is fine at home." Keep answers short and generic as much as possible.

They may ask about you looking tired, and you tell them you were up with your kid all night in the hospital. The patient then feels sorry for you (very kind of them). However, now that patient is worried about you. He or she is concerned about your feelings, and they feel bad if they "bother" you with stuff. So, they don't want to press the call light if they are in pain.

I have had patients say or ask me things that were really socially inappropriate. "How much money do you make?" Or "I think that other nurse likes me, what do you think my chances are with her?" Or "Do you hate (insert president here) as much as I do?" Or "They need to send those (insert race here) back to where they came from." These things can be very insulting, frustrating, and infuriating to the nurse.

Obviously, never let them drag you down that road of conversation. I usually tried to promptly turn the conversation back around to make them the focus... immediately. "Enough about me, let's talk about you. How is that pain medication doing for your back pain? Do we need to do another round of it?" (All said with a smile)

Also, "bar rules" apply. Do not engage in conversations about politics or religion. If they have political opinions different from yours, you don't have to agree with them, but you will never tell them you disagree. Avoid political conversations altogether if possible. Be kind and accepting of all races, religions, social statuses, sexual orientations, gender orientations, personal beliefs and practices, customs, and general personal preferences. Also recognize that you may not get the same courtesy in return. Believe it or not, people are racist (big surprise there, right? Ha!). That should not be a shock. I have seen patients (mostly really old and grumpy people) who refuse to be taken care of by anybody but a white person. I have seen patients of all ethnicity's who demand somebody of their same ethnicity take care of them. Anything can set a patient off. I have seen patients ask for a different nurse because they had trouble understanding an accent. You will meet all types.

I had a nurse under me in the ICU who was a very advanced and highly skilled cardiac nurse, who specialized in taking care of critically ill heart surgery patients. I used to say that if one of my family members was sick, she would be the nurse I would want to take care of them. However... she was totally incompetent socially. She had a strong accent and made no effort to provide clearer communication. She would break many of these rules... walk into rooms without knocking and start doing stuff, not explain things to the patient and family, be abrupt and "stand-offish," become easily frustrated and show it, and often show little compassion or patience.

However, if you needed a nurse to operate all of the life-support machines, and all of the medications, and all of the other devices, whose knowledge and ability to interpret advanced hemodynamic monitoring was beyond that of most nurses, and who always knows what to do, she was the one. If you wanted somebody kept alive who was otherwise collapsing medically, she was the nurse to assign to the case.

I occasionally would get called into a room to talk to a patient or family who had concerns about this particular nurse. I would tell them something similar to what I just told you. "I know she is rough around the edges, and I apologize for that, but I assure you she is the best at what she does, and medically speaking, you could not be in better hands." This would usually resolve the situation immediately.

This brings me to a final thought in this realm. Do your very best, at all times, to have clear communication with your patient. Explain what you are doing. Answer their questions. Ask permission to do things. Show confidence in yourself. Find ways to instill trust.

The safest thing is to leave your problems in the car, maintain a professional approach, do not let your facial expressions or body language communicate something negative, and do not tell patients details about your life or problems.

Keep the noise and laughter down at the nurse station.

I used to work with a couple of nurses who were notoriously loud when together. It was like they fed off each other, and the louder one laughed, the louder the other got. I could hear them from clear across the unit. I know the patients could hear them too. It's an ICU for God's sake. Patients should not be listening to nurses talk loud and joke and laugh in the hall. It should be a place of respect and quiet reverence.

These common sense practices can easily slip over time as you become desensitized to the job. A conscious effort will be required to keep yourself in check.

# Chapter 14:   Death and Dying

This portion of the book is a little long, but I think it is very important. It ends up being a major topic with which nurses will deal regularly, and it is a great opportunity to really provide care and comfort to the dying patient and their family. Further, I think the sorts of considerations that go along with working with the dying patient and their family can span into so many other areas of practice. If you can master this process, you can take care of patients and families with care and compassion in basically any setting. So, this setting serves as a good place to practice those skills.

Death can be a troubling subject for many new nurses. Many people have never actually touched a dead body before. Or maybe they have only ever seen a couple of deceased bodies in the context of a funeral home. They have a fear of this simple concept, as if something is different. They are fine touching the living body, but then upon death, the same physical body becomes scary, or repulsive, or creepy. Perhaps they can't even define it. They just feel weird about touching it. Maybe it's a product of modern television and movies, which glorify fictional concepts, like the "zombie." But it's important to remember, it's the same body. It may take time for some nurses to become comfortable with this aspect of care. Try to be prepared and anticipate how you will handle these things. The same goes for seeing blood, guts, and gore. In the ER, the deceased body may be in horrible shape. Depending on where you work, it's part of the job.

An obvious part of hospital life is dealing with death, and patients who are dying.

As always, I am no expert, but I will speak out of my experience. Modern American culture seems to have not really approached the concept of dying as being an expected part of life. We all know it happens, and we all know it will happen to us. But we don't like to talk about it. There is nothing secret or special about it. We all know exactly what it is. What happens after remains a mystery, and there are a thousand different beliefs.

**Resuscitation and CPR**

Sometimes it seems as though non-medical people assume that we fight to the very end for every patient. That every person who is dying will have CPR done on them. That we will never give up the battle until the doctor "calls it" in a dramatic fashion. This assumption is not made by everybody, but I have seen it many times among non-medical people. In reality, the vast majority of patients die in a smooth, predictable, and peaceful way, as we allow it to happen naturally and with medications to ensure comfort.

I have a good example. This was a case I worked in the ER. A woman was brought into the ER who was 102 years old. She was very sick with pneumonia. Her blood pressure was tanking, her heart rate was elevated, her blood work was terrible, and she looked equally as bad. Any attempt to get her through the illness would require extreme measures with low probability of success. She was going to be requiring a ventilator, vaso-active medications to support her blood pressure, and a whole river of IV antibiotics. Her kidneys would probably be failing quickly, and she would need immediate dialysis, among many other signs of critical illness. If left untreated, she had maybe a day, or maybe two. If treated, she would be put through lots of painful processes.

Upon seeing all of the data, the ER physician approached the patient's daughter, who was clearly up in her years as well by that point, considering their mother was 102.

The doctor stated the obvious, that the patient was probably going to die, even if we attempted aggressive treatment. He suggested that we consider palliative care. The immediate response from the (elderly) daughter was something like, "oh no, we have to fight for her, I can't lose my mom."

I don't have to explain the obvious to you. She was over 100, which is extremely rare. She was deathly ill. By most standards she had already beat the odds to make it that far. What was the daughter's expectation, that we would heal her mother and she would live to be 110? Of course, it is a dramatic and emotion-driven situation, so we can forgive some of the unrealistic expectations. People are not usually thinking straight in moments of loss and grief.

Most of the time, the scenarios are not that extreme. However, what we do constantly see in the ICU is a patient who, again, is deathly ill, and is getting worse every day. We keep increasing the life-support measures, and the patient continues to decline. Nothing we do can stop the coming collapse. In some of these cases, the family or patient may actually keep themselves as "full-code." This means that if (or when) they suffer cardiac and/or respiratory arrest, we will do CPR, and we will do everything possible to try and save their life, even though we know the efforts will be futile. The physician will even tell the family that when cardiac arrest occurs, if we try CPR, there is virtually a zero percent chance of success, and even if we are successful, it will happen again repeatedly until death. But the family wishes to continue the fight as long as possible, even through these events.

I had a physician who used to use the phrase, "We're just rearranging the deck chairs on the Titanic." The metaphor here, in case you don't get it, is that we are working tirelessly to keep this patient alive. We keep changing tests and treatments and medications and machines. We are making every effort to correct the problems as fast as they come, although we are falling behind. So, like the famous Titanic cruise ship from long ago, the boat is sinking. No matter how much we keep rearranging the deck chairs, the boat is still going down. It's a bit of a cold statement, but was only said among staff members in discussing expected outcomes. It would never be said in front of a patient or family.

I will not try to quote statistics, but the reality is that only a small percentage of CPR cases actually save the patient's life. On TV, they can always keep going and if they just shock enough times, the patient will survive. Then the patient wakes up and feels great, as if they were just sleeping. A real patient who survives CPR has been pulled back from the brink of death, but that does not mean they are not still standing right next to the brink. If the injury or illness is so bad that it causes cardiac and/or respiratory arrest, the likelihood of another crash is extremely high. Successful CPR did not fix the original problem that caused it in the first place. So, a very small percentage of medical patients are successfully kept alive by CPR. "Medical" means that the cause is an underlying non-traumatic disease process in the body, like heart failure, sepsis, or blood clotting problems leading to internal bleeding. Out of those few who survive, a very small percentage will ever leave the hospital alive, as more crashes are to come. If the arrest is caused by trauma (rather than a medical cause), the chances of CPR working are almost zero.

There are exceptions to this rule. Sometimes an acute situation can occur, causing an arrest and requiring CPR, but the underlying single cause can be fixed. This would be like an otherwise healthy person suddenly having a heart attack that caused arrest. The arrest is witnessed and CPR is started immediately. Or perhaps an electrolyte level, like potassium suddenly becomes so high or low that it causes a change in the EKG rhythm. With advanced cardiac life support measures, the patient is kept alive by artificial means. And in a short time we have corrected the electrolyte imbalance medically, or they are in the cath lab where an interventional cardiologist is able to open the blocked coronary artery, thereby restoring blood flow to that portion of the heart. There may be some damage done to their heart from lack of blood flow, and there may even be some damage done to the brain from insufficient blood flow. But, with successful resuscitation and with a successful cath lab procedure or other immediately-curative intervention, there is a very high likelihood that the patient will survive.

Another exception might be drowning. An otherwise healthy person who drowns, if caught quickly, might be resuscitated. There have also been cases where a person drowns in extremely cold water, and are successfully resuscitated after a very long period of being "down" (without a heart beat), and actually recover with little or no brain damage. In the ICU after patients are resuscitated, we put them into therapeutic hypothermia, which means we artificially cool their body down well below the normal body temperature. This reduces metabolism and cell activity, and will preserve neurological function as the body is recovering from being in cardiac arrest. So the freezing water drowning is a similar concept.

Also, patients who have had a heart procedure, like open heart surgery, have a higher tendency to have a cardiac arrest because the heart is acutely ill and irritated from being messed with. But these patients are already on all of the life support machines and medications as they are recovering from the surgery. So, we often times do not even have to start CPR. If we see they suddenly switch into a rhythm that is shockable by a defibrillator, like ventricular tachycardia, ventricular fibrillation, unstable atrial fibrillation, or unstable supraventricular tachycardia, everything is in place, including the defibrillator (from being in surgery), and so we just start shocking. Of, course, we will start compressions if a pulse is fully lost. It works most of the time. All of the other necessary cardiac medications to treat the sick heart are already in place, and the patient is already on a ventilator, so this is successful most of the time.

On that subject, television tends to misrepresent what a diffibrillator does. The patient is in "asystole," which is commonly called "flat-lining" on television. By the way, never say "flat-lining" for real when working as a nurse. People will laugh at you. "Asystole" is the correct term. With asystole, or "flat line," there is no electrical activity flowing through the cardiac tissue to initiate a mechanical response by the muscles, causing a beat of the heart. The television medical personnel will begin to repeatedly difibrillate the patient, as if the shock is going to restart a dead "flat-lined" heart. In reality, this is far from the truth. Shocking the heart does not "restart" it like on television. Difribrillation, in the most simplistic terms possible, basically stops the heart (by a complex series of biological mechanisms), allowing the normal electrical signal pathway to restart again. It's like rebooting a computer. Shocking a "flat-line" heart does not help. Instead, CRP and ACLS medications are provided, which may help the heart to restore its own electrical activity, and then shocks may be required to fix the rhythm. There are also different types of shocks. A difibrillator may be used for actual "defibrillation" for some rhythms, or can be used for "synchronized cardioversion" for some rhythms, or and can be used as a temporary emergency external pacemaker. I have used it for all of these many, many, many times. Oh, and one last thing. The patient does not arch up dramatically in the bed. Their body usually just makes a little jerking motion. And, there is no sound. Sorry, the "clear....WHAM!" on television does not happen. But we do say "clear."

So, a patient is by default classified as a "full code,"

meaning that everything possible will be tried to keep them alive if they arrest. The opposite of that is the "do not resuscitate" order, or "DNR." DNR gets bad publicity, as people often view is as meaning "do not treat." This is not the case. There are many different scenarios that use a DNR order. In most cases, DNR means that we will do everything we can to keep a person alive, but at the moment their heart stops or they stop breathing, we will not do compressions nor will we place them on a ventilator. We might even still give advanced cardiac life support medications. Just no CPR.

Many older people like to be classified as a DNR, as they know that if they are sick enough to arrest, an attempt to resuscitate them will have poor odds. Plus, if they are resuscitated, there is a high likelihood that they will be reliant on life support measures indefinitely to keep them alive. Many people just don't want that. They don't want to end up in a long-term acute care facility with a permanent ventilator and a tracheostomy, and a surgically implanted feeding tube in their stomach, and where they will spend the remainder of their days in pain and in a bed hooked to machines. But DNR patients do continue to receive aggressive curative therapy as long as they have not arrested. They will have surgeries, receive all the same medications and antibiotics, and will otherwise be treated just like any other "full-code" patient.

In a case of palliative care, a patient will have to be made a DNR, as it is known they are going to be allowed to die naturally. They can't be both "full-code" and have a palliative care plan. In these cases, aggressive curative measures are not attempted.

The in-between case is the "full-code" who has gone so far downhill that they are not expected to live much longer, even with aggressive treatments. They are going to die either way. They are dependent on ventilators and medications and other machines. When it is apparent that

203

curative measures have failed, the family may opt to "withdraw care." This simply means the patient will be changed to DNR status, and all life support measures will be removed, including the ventilator and medications, and other devices if being used. In this case, the patient usually dies withing minutes, or maybe a few hours. Meanwhile, they will be given generous doses of pain medication to ensure they are comfortable.

## Palliative Care

As previously mentioned, the intent of palliative care is to focus all efforts on comfort rather than cure. In some cases, the patient will live for a long time on palliative care, maybe six months or longer. In other cases, the patient may last days or weeks.

Under palliative care standards, the patient will not receive any medications, except for those that promote comfort and quality of life. They will have no painful procedures or treatments. They will not get their blood drawn constantly. There are always exceptions to these rules. Sometimes a palliative care patient may have a surgery done to provide comfort. Perhaps they have a tumor or cancerous mass removed. It is understood that this will not prolong life, and the cancer will still end their life, but the tumor was pressing on an organ or on the spine, or in some way causing pain. In some cases, the patient or family may like to continue to have vital signs checked occasionally, or have finger-sticks done to check blood sugar levels. There are limitless possibilities.

Some palliative care patients will go to the other extreme, where absolutely nothing is done, and they are basically given enough pain medicine to keep them unconscious until they die, which may take hours, days, or maybe a week.

Hospice is a well-known palliative care organization.

I have worked in hospitals that had an actual Hospice inpatient unit, and have worked on one of those units. All patients there were under palliative care. The rooms looked like hotel rooms, with pictures and nice walls, and even normal-looking furniture. All medical devices, like oxygen and suction valves attached to the walls are hidden behind cabinet doors. The actual bed might even be a normal-looking bed, instead of a hospital bed. They have nice sheets and pillows and blankets. If you were to wake up in a Hospice room like this, and did not know where you were, you would not know it was a hospital room. The environment is kept quiet, there is peaceful music available if desired, a really nice waiting room with real furniture, and the constant presence of clergy or chaplains. It's a really awesome experience to work there. There has always been a special place in my heart for palliative care, and I enjoyed doing it.

In some cases, a Hospice patient lives in a nursing home, or even in their home with a care-giver. In these cases, there will be a Hospice case worker, generally an RN, who will do daily visits to these patients and families, and who will be on call for emergencies or to pronounce death. They have the authority to change medication and treatment orders as needed to promote comfort, without the presence of a physician. And, of course, there are dedicated palliative care doctors.

**Advanced Directives**

An advanced directive is a legal document created by a person while they are still healthy and of sound mind, which will direct exactly how they want their care to be handled if or when they are not conscious or are in any way mentally altered beyond the ability to make important medical decisions. These are really good as they take the burden of heavy decisions off of the family. It may say that the patient desires to be a "full-code," but in the case they are revived and it is evident they will be dependent on life support measures permanently, they wish for care to be withdrawn. I have seen that example many times.

It might say that they do not ever want a feeding tube implanted. Or it might just direct the physician to change them to DNR status if they become incapacitated beyond decision-making ability. There are numerous possibilities.

With the medical technology we have to artificially keep people alive, we have now begun to create a new challenge in medicine. There was a time long ago when a major heart attack was lethal, as there were no defibrillators, cardiac medications, and cath labs. There was no life-support machines to decide whether or not to use. Before antibiotics, a simple cut on the finger could become infected, and lead to septic shock and death. In those times, perhaps the concepts of DNR versus full-code did not exist, at least not the way we see them today.

There are ethical and philosophical questions that come from all of this. One might say that by artificially keeping people alive, we are "playing god" by prolonging life when nature would have already taken the life. On the other hand, if we have the technology, but choose not to use it, are we "playing god" by allowing people to die when we have the capacity to keep them alive a little longer. Where is the line drawn between wanting to extend life as far as possible, no matter now much suffering there is, versus making a decision to allow the dying process to happen and accept that while treatment might keep the person alive, the suffering would outweigh the quality of life. It's the question of quality versus quantity. If you are really hungry, would you rather have a lot of pizza that tastes terrible, or would you rather have the best pizza in existence, but only get one slice? Would you rather die comfortably in one week? Or would you rather live six more months, but spend that time in the

206

hospital hooked to machines and having painful things done to you constantly?

The ethical and philosophical questions surrounding these topics can go on forever. However, in real-life application, there is rarely a single moment when a patient goes from possibly curable, to terminal with imminent death. That would make decisions a lot easier if the doctor could come in and say, "We got the death test back. The patient is going to live only three more days."

While it becomes somewhat obvious to medical professionals how cases are going to turn out, it still puts difficult questions on the patient and family. In the absence of an advanced directive, an unconscious patient may have different family members arguing for different paths in care. One wants comfort care, and the other wants to sustain life as long as possible. Which one is correct? That question generally comes down to a legal matter of who has the authority to make the decision. Further, even if the family is all in agreement, there still comes a time when they must decide for themselves that curative care should be stopped. They will make their decision, but then spend the rest of their life wondering if it was the right decision. "Maybe she would have pulled through if we had just waited a little longer..." Or, "Why did we wait so long to stop care, and let her suffer so much..." This is a serious burden to be placed on family members.

Finally, there are always the outlying cases when a person survives against all odds, or dies in a sudden and unexpected manner. In modern medicine, with our advanced capabilities, death is now something we have to negociate with, not just work against.

**Types of Death**

Death can come in many forms. A gunshot or car wreck causing trauma to the brain may introduce instant death. A patient may be awake and collapse on the floor due to cardiac arrest, because of a sudden heart attack or stroke. Sometimes a patient may have a heart attack or stroke, and die over the course of a day as their heart or brain are slowly overwhelmed by the damage done. However, most people will die slowly. It is not an event. It is a process. There are complex set of changes that occur in the body over time as it dies.

A common scene on television is the guy who has been shot, or who is critically ill, and they are awake, coherent, and speaking to someone. And then, mid-sentence, they suddenly stop talking and their head falls to the side. Their skin was nice and pink, or normal color for whatever race. They have no confusion or disorientation. They are wide awake and tuned into the world and they don't look bad at all, and then their head drops while talking and that's it. Perfectly living and functioning brain, to dead brain in an instant, and without additional trauma to cause that instant to occur. It's a great dramatic death for television, but I have never seen one in real life. And I have seen a lot of deaths.

Perhaps something similar may happen to a person who has been shot and is rapidly bleeding enough to very suddenly become unconscious from lack of oxygen to the brain. It might be something that is more commonly seen by the military with violent combat-related deaths. I will not pretend to know. So, maybe something similar has happened out there, but I doubt it happens very often, and it would be especially and exceedingly rare in the hospital setting, and basically non-existent in the case of a medical patient dying.

In fact, the exact moment of "death" is not always clearly defined in a patient who is dying slowly and naturally.

**The Dying Process**

Let's take a hypothetical patient, who is elderly, very sick, and is going into septic shock, or cardiogenic shock, or any number of the other shocks. Death will be imminent in the absence of aggressive life-supporting care. But in this case, the patient or family has chosen palliative care. The patient may be awake for a while. However, as time goes on, they will often become confused, lethargic, and will eventually slip into an unconscious state (slowly). This part of the process may take days or even a week. It's usually not fast.

As time passes, kidney and liver failure will result in alterations in fluid and electrolyte balance, along with blood pH, essentially making the blood toxic. Insufficient breathing will further cause the blood to become dangerously acidic. As these sorts of changes happen, the ability to regain consciousness is lost, and multi-system organ failure is in full progression.

Now that the patient is unconscious, or comatose, or whatever you want to call it, you will begin to see objective signs of the body "shutting down." Urine output will slow and maybe stop completely as the kidneys shut down over a day or two. The patient will become less responsive to pain or stimuli, and might not react at all. Meaning, you might pinch their skin hard enough to cause pain, and get no physical reaction. They will be completely immobile, and generally will take on a flaccid posture, meaning their body is basically fully limp. With this, their mouth will tend to hang fully open. Their eye lids may be closed, or may hang open, and can usually be manipulated in either way.

They will have a fixed gaze, meaning the pupils do not move around as if looking or seeing. A common reflex we check is the "dolls eyes" reflex.

So, let's do a quick demonstration. You, the reader, look straight ahead at the wall. Now, begin to turn your head from side to side and continue looking at the same spot on the wall. This should come very easy and without conscious effort. This is a reflex that keeps the eyes fixed on a point while the head moves around them. Now, look straight forward, and turn your head side to side again. But this time, make your eyes move with your turning head, as you look straight forward, and your gaze moves with your head. You will notice that it requires conscious effort to make your eyes do this. I hope that makes sense. A dying patient will at some point lose this reflex. If you gently turn their head from side to side, their eyes and gaze will remain fixed and move with their head.

You may note that their pupils become dilated, fixed, and unresponsive to light. Normally, when you shine a light in a patient's eyes, the pupils will constrict as a reflex to the increased light. It's exactly what happens when you leave the house and go into the sun, and everything is too bright for a moment until your eyes adjust.

There are numerous other reflexes that can be checked, and you will begin to see these reflexes slow and even stop in the dying patient.

Cheyne-Stokes respirations can be a sign of impeding pulmonary failure. These are characterized by periods of taking breaths on regular intervals and then abruptly or slowly begin to not breathe, and after a short period of apnea, the patient will take a large gasping breath, and the cycle repeats. This is very similar to what happens to patients with sleep apnea. With this breathing pattern can also come pharyngeal rales. This is also commonly referred to as a "death rattle," although medical professionals would certainly refrain from using the latter term in front of patients or families. This presents as a perpetual rattling or gurgling sound in the upper airway. It is pretty unmistakable. The instinct for an alert person would be to choke, cough, gag, and clear their throat in the presence of secretion build-up in the back of the throat and upper airways. But the patient is now unconscious to the point that no reflexive airway clearance activity occurs.

Mottling is commonly believed to be a sign of imminent death in most patients. Imminent death does not mean immediately, but means death is approaching, and will occur in the coming hours or days, or possibly even a week or more. It is not a question of "if," but a question of "when." This is characterized by the skin of the outer extremities changing color. In a lighter-skinned patient, it is very easy to see. Disorganized patches or blotches of red, purple, and blue will begin to cover the toes, feet, and legs, as it starts at the most distal point and slowly moves inward toward the center of the body. It may have a marbled appearance, and these blotches will have continuity. They are not patches among areas of normal healthy skin. The entirety of the skin is involved. This is also pretty unmistakable when it occurs. A simple internet search of the term "mottling skin" will turn up plenty of pictures.

Mottling is a result of the distal tissues becoming cyanotic, or as blood flow is no longer sufficient to the outer extremities to provide oxygenation. The toe nails will take on a deep blue or purple color, and capillary refill may be absent. This is the early stages of the tissues dying from lack of blood flow and oxygen. If the patient survives long enough, the skin may turn deep solid black and tight, resembling a mummy.

Once the patient is approaching the last minutes or hour before death, they may progress through changes on the EKG monitor quickly or slowly. In come cases, the heart rate takes on a steady downward trajectory over an hour. Eventually it will just be an occasionally bump on the EKG rhythm, and it will no longer be a traditionally-shaped EKG complex. It's just a bump, and is a sign of the heart making a final agonal effort to beat. After minutes of intermittent agonal beats, the EKG line will fall flat completely, with no further activity. Breaths may do the same, as the patient may go for 30 seconds or almost a minute without taking a breath, but then will suddenly take one small gasping breath. These EKG changes may also occur quickly over a minute or two. These are signs of the body making its final agonal efforts to sustain life.

The question remains. At what point during this process was the patient actually "dead?" Do we define it with a hard objective description, like the moment the EKG rhythm becomes permanently flat? Or the moment the last of the brain activity stops (which would require additional devices to monitor)? If there is a spirit or soul, does it leave the body before these events happen, or at those exact moments, or even after? This is less a medical question and more a philosophical question perhaps. In the hospital the pronouncement of death generally comes at the time the EKG rhythm is flat and no pulse, breath sounds, heart sounds, or pupil response can be detected, and all efforts for resuscitation have stopped.

After death, as the muscles and tissues relax, urine or stool may be passed, or may keep passing occasionally whenever the body is manipulated. A process called dependent lividity will commence. As the blood vessels lose tone, and there is no heart pumping blood, the blood will begin to flow through the vessels in a response to gravity. So the blood will all pool into the vessels in the bottom half of the patient. If the patient is lying flat, it will be seen in the back of the legs, the buttocks, the back, and the backs of the arms and hands. Meanwhile the upper body portions will become pale as they are drained of blood. The areas where the blood settles turn a deep purple. This is another pretty unmistakable phenomena. And, perhaps the more well-known process of rigor mortis sets in after a few hours, as the muscles begin to tense, and the body becomes rigid. These are generally the only parts of the process the nurse will witness. As I have said before, you can do an internet search for "dependant lividity pictures" and see for yourself what that looks like.

I have had cases, especially in the ER, when patients were continuously oozing frothy blood from their mouths or nose or other orifices. Something like this may happen, and will complicate your preparing the body for viewing. You get the blood cleaned and the mouth suctioned out and cleaned, and then it all starts flowing as soon as the body is moved even a little. A death in response to trauma, burn, or other physical injury may present its own complications. Obviously, severe facial trauma would be difficult to make viewable by a family.

**Family support and Post-Mortem Care**

The nurse's job does not end when the patient dies. There is still plenty of work to be done. Once a patient has been pronounced dead, the possible series of events can vary from extreme drama to peaceful closure, or anywhere in between.

In the more complex situations, especially if death was not expected, the whole scenario obviously catches the family by surprise. The patient may be in the emergency department, or maybe an inpatient unit. The family may be present, or at home, or may not even know the patient is in the hospital at all, in many cases of the ER. The ER physician will generally handle the job of communicating with a family of a patient who has died in an unexpected nature. This is especially intense when the patient was a baby, or child, or teenager, or young adult. Maybe the patient had very young children, and their surprised spouse is suddenly left alone. Or maybe there is no spouse, and the children are suddenly without a legal guardian as their single parent just died.

A common situation in the emergency department is the spontaneous abortion, or miscarriage. This is not the traditional abortion, whereby the mother decides to make it happen. This is the when the fetus has died or the body has another problem, leading to its early evacuation of the uterus. A semi-developed and deceased baby is passed from the mother. These are difficult moments for the mother and father. If it happens very early, it may just be heavy bleeding and no detectable fetus can be found. If later, the baby, at whatever stage of development, will be passed from the uterus. This can be just like having a newborn baby die for parents. The handling and final disposition of the fetus or premature baby might vary, and in some cases, a funeral and burial might occur. That is all up to the parents.

The mother experiencing the miscarriage may blame herself or otherwise experience extreme guilt, but in most cases, she had really done nothing wrong.

Entire volumes of books could be written on the phenomena of communicating with patient families after a death. The applicable psychology and philosophy concepts, and real-life consequences are innumerable.

Fortunately, the nurse is very rarely caught in the middle of these cases alone and without a physician. Nurses certainly have their part, but the higher medical authority of the physician generally shoulders the burden of providing news that is surprising to a patient or family. The nurse may not have to communicate the information, but they are still usually present to watch the drama unfold and assist according to their job, license, and scope of practice. After the initial shock occurs, family members generally have access to followup assistance and care for the short and long-term. Much of the care may come in the form of their own healthcare providers. The healthcare team includes all of the various professionals who can help families in these cases, including (but not limited to) clergy, psychologists, psychiatrists, therapists, case managers, social workers, and even funeral home staff. If Hospice was involved, that organization may have support mechanisms for family.

A more common death is the planned "withdrawal of care" or otherwise allowance of natural death on short notice. In these cases, the family should never be caught by surprise. They most often will be present when it happens, and will already have a full understanding of what is coming.

The competent nurse should be present to walk the family through the process. That may include providing education on the expected physiological changes that will be witnessed. As discussed earlier, the body changes that occur during death can be dramatic and might be disturbing to a family member who does not understand.

The nurse will remain present, or at least close-by, and ready to serve the family in any way needed. This is the time to turn on the ultra-professional and ultra-compassionate nurse inside you. Speak quietly, no joking, no laughing, no fast or rough movements, extra gentle, extra slow, extra patient, extra generous, smile in a caring and loving way, ensure that the hall space outside the room is kept quiet, provide for gentle lighting the room... Let your fellow nurses and staff know that you have a patient dying with family at the bedside, so they will be extra diligent to avoid making noise in the area. I've been hugged by patient family members during and after the process, and on countless occasions I have held the hand of the patient at the time they die. This last part was just something meaningful to me. If there was lots of family, I would encourage them to circle the bed and hold the patient's hands, and I would remain in the background. However, if the family was absent, I liked to be present, just so the patient had "somebody" there.

I won't get off into philosophies or religious beliefs or metaphysical concepts or fringe science. However, we don't understand what happens after death. Maybe the soul remains in the body and aware for a while. Maybe the soul leaves the body but remains briefly present. Maybe the mind comprehends more than we know. Maybe the patient knows their hand is being held before they die. Maybe speaking to the recently deceased body as post-mortem care is provided gives comfort to the freshly celestially-released spirit. Maybe the presence of a caring person somehow helps the patient smoothly and peacefully transition from this life to the next. Or, maybe it makes no difference at all and is totally unnecessary. But, just to be on the safe side, I like to be there to provide the presence of a peaceful, loving, and nurturing person as the patient finishes this chapter of the life cycle. It certainly could not hurt. And, of course, if the patient has family, but they are not present when it happens, it's awesome to get to tell them *you* were their and held the patient's hand, and ensured that it was easy, painless, and peaceful. Families tend to be eternally grateful that you were there, and the patient was not alone.

If the patient's family is present, the nurse will generally do the initial notification of death. If the family is not present, but the death is anticipated, the nurse will generally call the family for the notification. In the ICU, I would be outside watching the heart monitor, and could see when cardiac electrical activity comes to a complete stop. I would enter the room, gently and reverently check pupil response to light, check for a pulse, and listen for breath or heart sounds with a stethoscope. Usually the family could already tell the patient was dead. It usually looks quite obvious. But this is the proper way to finish the process with concern and care, when in the presence of the family. Again, the family usually knew at that point, but they would look to me for expert confirmation.

After my assessment, I would then look up with a modest and reverent smile, and simply say that he/she had passed. Maybe let your eyes go from person to person, and make brief eye contact with each individual who is still looking at you. It's like acknowledging their presence once more, and letting them know that while you are speaking to the room, you are also speaking to them individually. It's one of those old nursing tricks.

The doctor would be paged to come by and pronounce. They often did not arrive for a while as it is not urgent. The nurse notes the time of death, and the doctor uses that time. If the family is present, the doctor will offer their own kind words, and may very well do the same assessment of the eyes, pulse, and breath sounds, although they know it is not necessary.

Once the patient is deceased, the family will look to the nurse for the next steps. The process is usually simple. There will often be just one or two pages of paperwork to fill out, and signed by the family if they are present. It includes things like an inventory of the patient's personal belongings in the room. If the family has selected a funeral home, that information can be noted also. And contact information for the family members is also listed. If possible, it is fine to allow the family to have ample time with the body. They do not need to be hurried from the room. Unless the room is urgently needed for another critical patient, here is no hurry for anything. At some point, the nurse will call the funeral home, or an on-call pickup service, and the representative will eventually show up to take the body. Or, the nurse will take the body to a cooler until it can be picked up later. The family may or may not still be present by that time. The nurse will still have plenty of documentation to be done on the patient.

There are limitless little nuances in the process, and the process may be different in varying facilities. But this gives the general idea.

But there are a few key things to learn out of this. You are <u>not</u> a philosopher. You are <u>not</u> exceedingly wise. You do <u>not</u> have insight into the workings of the astral realm. It is totally *inappropriate* for you to make trite comments as a show of support. For example, <u>never say</u>...

217

"He's in God's hands now."
"He's dancing with the angels now."
"God took him home."
"He fought so hard."
"He's in a better place."
"His suffering is over."
"I know he must have been a good man."
"Rest in peace, old friend."
"Your healing can start now" (talking to the family)

The family may make these statements, but you should not. If they do, you may agree with them in some way, but will not offer further thoughts. If the wrong thing is said by the nurse, it can be frustrating or even maddening for the family. It is better to say too little than to say too much. A simple statement intended to help the family can unintentionally cause great harm.

You may say...
"I'm so sorry for your loss."
"I am here for anything you need."
"Please take your time and just be with him/her if you like."
"Can I bring you coffee/water/etc?"
"Would you like to be left alone and have some privacy or would you like me to stay for a while?"
"If there is anything special you would like us to do for Mr. /Mrs. Doe, please tell me, and I will be happy to assist."

And, a very important detail to remember... Always continue to refer to the body as "Mr. or Mrs. Doe," especially in front of the family. Do not tell the family "the funeral home will pick up the body." Tell them, the funeral home will pick up "Mrs. Doe." Maintain the humanity and dignity of the person. It's not just a body. It's still a loved member of a grieving family. And, even after death, the person is still "your patient." You will continue to treat the physical body with respect and dignity. You will not unnecessarily expose the body, just like when giving a bath. Keep things covered with towels. Keep the curtains and door closed. As always, treat the body the way you would want the body of your family members treated, regardless of whether anyone is watching.

The actual post-mortem care of the body will vary depending on the presence or absence of the family, the condition of the body, the presence of infectious diseases, and the presence of external machines or devices. You will check your hospital policy about what to remove and what to leave in place. If there is to be an autopsy ordered, they will probably prefer that the breathing tube be left in place, and perhaps any sort of central intravenous catheters or dialysis ports. It may be best to leave the urinary catheter in place too. These things can all be easily removed by the funeral home. Again, check your hospital policy on items regarding law-enforcement notification of a death, determining if autopsy is to be performed, and technical matters on preparing and labeling the body.

I did have cases where a patient suddenly became very sick at home, was taken to the ER, placed on life-support mechanisms, and then promptly died within 24 hours. 99.9% of the time, it is probably a totally natural process that occurred. However, that is not your call to make. Some facilities want you to call the police for any patient that dies within the first 24 hours of hospitalization. I did this many times. They usually just made a quick report over the phone and nothing else ever happened. However, a couple of times, they instructed me to not touch the body any more, including no post-mortem care, and that a detective will come to the hospital. They show up and ask questions, and take the body into their custody. A funeral home usually still comes to pick the body up, but they then work with the police to maintain and store the body in a way that is appropriate for an autopsy. Again, check you hospital protocols.

If you are working in the emergency department, and

a death is caused by violence, you absolutely should not manipulate or clean the body in any way. Things like gunshot residue may be present on the skin, and should not be washed away. Perhaps there is blood under the finger nails from scratching the attacker. Maybe there is semen around the vaginal opening, in case a sexual assault came with a murder. Think of all the possible DNA evidence that could be ruined if the body is washed.

Some general things that are usually safe to do are to wash the body (unless law enforcement instructs not to), to a greater or lesser extent. Place a fresh clean gown without wrinkles on the body. Center the body in the bed. Any medical devices still attached should be tucked under the blanket. The bed should have fresh clean sheets and blankets. The top sheet and blanket may be pulled up to the patient's chest, and the edge folded back down on itself, making a nice sharp clean line. The sheet/blanket should reach up to just below the level of the armpits. The arms can then be taken from under the covers and placed on top, and positioned neatly at the patient's sides. Then raise the head of the bed slightly, maybe 20 degrees. This leaves the patient clean, fresh, cleared of blood or urine or stool, with clean sheets that cover the body up to the chest level. The arms and hands are exposed to allow the family the ability to touch and hold. A pillow can be placed behind the head to help provide support for better positioning. Ultimately, this will all make the patient look "comfortable," thereby making viewing easier and more pleasant. The eye lids can usually be pulled closed. The mouth usually will not close.

Remove all equipment possible from the room. IV pumps and poles, bags of IV medications hanging, monitoring equipment, loose hoses or wires or tubes, any medical device that is removed or detached from the body... Set the lighting in the room to be peaceful. In my ICU, there was a fluorescent light positioned on the wall above the head of the bed. The fixture was only open to the top, and completely opaque on the front and bottom, so it provided a less-bright pleasant indirect light to the room. Having dim light might make physiological changes in the body look less dramatic. Think of if you have ever done a viewing in a state room of a funeral home. The room lighting is usually kept dim and indirect. Make sure all other overhead lighting is off. Clean up clutter, organize anything left in the room, empty all trash cans, etc.

Keep the curtains closed, and the door closed to ensure privacy for the family. Make the environment as peaceful as possible. Sometimes the unit may have a special sign or sticker to place on the door. We had a little picture of a dove flying in front of a sunset, about the size of a post card. It said "peace be with you," or something like that below the bird. We would tape it to the door. It is small and attracts very little attention. But it notifies any staff who come along about what is happening. Maybe house keeping shows up to empty trash. Maybe a new CNA shows up on the unit to help out. Maybe dietary shows up to drop off a dinner tray. This will prevent awkward situations of someone trying to perform normal operations in the middle of this dramatic moment immediately after death.

Please do not let the family show up and the patient looks disheveled, and/or be covered in blood/stool/urine/etc, and still be hooked to IV lines and monitoring equipment. If the family is present at the time of death, and then promptly leaves, extensive aesthetic post-mortem care may not be necessary. Or the family may like to step out while you do these things, and then come back to be with the body. If the family is not present at all, has to be called for notification, and they are going to come to the hospital... Do everything you can to make that body look as good as possible before they show up. And, in general, you usually do not need to cover the head with a sheet like they do on television.

# Chapter 15:   Hard Days & Situations

**Frustrations**

Consider a scenario where an elderly patient is critically ill, and hope for meaningful recovery is lost. Perhaps the daughter wants to withdraw care and allow the patient to pass.   The daughter had been designated on a medical power of attorney, by the patient, to have the legal authority to make these decisions if the patient were incapacitated.   However, the patient's son shows up.   He demands that care continue.   Technically, he does not have the legal authority to make that decision.   If the daughter overrules him, and care is withdrawn, he may feel like his sister and the hospital "killed" or even "murdered" his parent.

In some cases, the daughter may even make a decision that the son should receive no information regarding the patient.   Further, if he shows up to the hospital, her instructions are that he is not allowed to see the patient, nor can the hospital even acknowledge the patient is present.  She has that legal authority, just as if the patient were awake, and could instruct the hospital to keep the patient anonymous and allow no visitors.

The son: "Hi, I'm here to see Mr. Doe, my father."

The ICU nurse: "I'm sorry, I don't see anyone by that name on my list."

The son: "I know he's here.  I just talked to my sister, but she said I wasn't supposed to come see him, but I don't care, I want to see him anyway."

The ICU nurse: "I'm sorry sir, I do not have anybody by that name listed as a patient."

The son: (now angry) "I know good-and-damn-well that he is here.  And I know my sister probably told you not to tell me.

I'm so pissed at her, but I'll deal with her later. Now, where is he?"

The ICU nurse: "I'm sorry sir...

You can see how the exchange can become heated quickly. The daughter has the legal right to make the patient anonymous in the hospital, as far as confirming or denying the patient's presence. In this case, yes, the son knows the patient is present. Are you allowed to acknowledge the patient's presence? No. Can the nurse say, "Look, I know that you know the patient is here, but I'm not allowed to acknowledge it."? No. Can the nurse say, "I can't tell you where the patient is, but if you just want to look around you'll probably find them (wink wink)."? No.

This is a nasty place in which to get caught when dealing with patients' families. I have been there many times. How does this scenario resolve over time? Does the son shrug his shoulders and decide he was mistaken and peacefully walk away with no further questions or concerns? Of course not.

Does the nurse finally say, "Sir, I have this list in my hands. It has names on it of the patients in the hospital. If the name is not on the list, I can't acknowledge that the patient is here. Whether the patient is somewhere and being kept anonymous, and therefore is not on my list... well, I have no idea, because I just have my list."?

Maybe this makes the son realize the situation and understand your position, and brings a more peaceful resolution. You let on that the patient is there, you just can't say where. But did you do the right thing? No. You gave just enough of a clue to confirm the patient's presence, but without actually making the clear statement and acknowledgment. That still conflicts with the daughter's legal instructions.

Perhaps the nurse finally says, "Sir, I realize your frustration in looking for your parent. I'm afraid I just don't

223

have any information that will be helpful to you. Perhaps you should call your sister and discuss with her where the patient might be, and what his/her current condition is." This might be a little more on track to maintain your obligations, while deflecting the son's attack away from yourself.

But, meanwhile, the sister should be made aware that it's not appropriate for the nurse to have to be caught in the middle of a family dispute of this nature. If she doesn't want the son to know where the parent is, then she needs to tell him that. Don't say the patient is here, and then shift the burden onto the nurses to protect his/her privacy. If she wants to tell the son that the parent is in the hospital, but she has instructed the staff to keep the location secret, then the nurse can say, "I'm sorry sir, I have been instructed by the patient's daughter to not disclose the location." At least then, you are not acting like you don't even know if the patient is present.

How far does it go? Does the son get frustrated and leave? Does he keep fighting and getting increasingly angry? Do you eventually call security to remove him from the building because he is making a scene?

I wish I could tell you there was a simple answer. In any heated situation like this, all you have to do is "a," then "b," then "c." And the situation will resolve itself, and the angry family member will be happy and hug you.

Unfortunately, many scenarios in healthcare have no "right" answer. We just have to find the answer that minimizes risk to a patient, ensures safety of the staff, and minimizes any legal exposure the organization might have. People love threatening to sue a hospital. I never cared to hear that mess. I would just tell the person I would make a note of it and send an e-mail to the risk management department and to my manager and/or director. Otherwise, I did not listen to, or acknowledge threats, beyond just saying "I will pass that along."

**Tragedies**

I had a difficult case, in which a man with mental health problems (in his late 20's or early 30's) had locked himself away in a hotel room, without his family knowing his whereabouts. He drank and exceedingly large amount of alcohol, and took a whole bottle of Tylenol. He was found passed out the next day by the housekeeping staff. If he had been found earlier, we might have been able to give medications to protect his liver from the Tylenol overdose. But, as hours had passed, the damage was done. He was quickly moved into the ICU, in profound acute liver failure. His skin glowed bright yellow from the buildup of bilirubin in his blood, as is expected with a hepatic patient. His stools were yellow and pasty and had a very high-pitch odor from the bilirubin his body was dumping. The blood clotting factors that are normally managed by the liver were dysfunctional, so he was internally bleeding. We just kept transfusing blood and blood products with clotting factors, but it's never enough.

His ammonia level was critical high, and his blood was essentially toxic in every way imaginable in the absence of hepatic filtration. A patient can't live very long like this. With failed kidneys, a patient can be put on dialysis for years. There is no replacement device for the liver. The only possible hope for survival would have been a liver transplant. But, he was pretty much dying within a couple of days, and that was never going to happen. He was unconscious and on a ventilator, so he had no idea what was going on around him. It was a very sad case.

But, it gets even sadder. His young wife brought their two kids (both under the age of 10) up to the ICU, so they could tell their Daddy goodbye. I had kids that same age when this case happened. Picturing my own children having to experience that type of pain made (and sill makes) me physically ill. That was a hard day for all of us. It's still painful for me to think about that case, years later. I sometimes think about those kids, and where they might be today, and how their lives have moved on. They will be damaged, there is no question about that. I cried about that one when it happened, and I could almost still do it now. I cried about a lot of cases. Never while at work, and never in front of anyone. But I would not be human if I had not been upset by so many things I saw.

I wish I could tell you this was the only horrible think I ever saw. But it wasn't. There was sadness around every corner...

## Cases That Intimately and Personally Disturb You

I've talked about seeing difficult things with kids in the ER. And, again, I have kids who were really young at the time. I remember often seeing my own kids' faces in the children with whom I worked. I had to make conscious efforts to push my kids out of my head while working sometimes. It's like a built-in mechanism, perhaps a protective parental process, whereby you see something so tragic and painful involving a child, and your first instinct is to imagine it happening to your own children, so you will try harder to protect them.

As a parent, one that always haunted me the most was when you hear of a baby being accidently left in a hot car. I always wondered how a person can go on living. It was not on purpose. People are not perfect. Accidents happen. The person who did it is not bad or evil. They are a regular person. But it's so unimaginably tragic that it's difficult to stretch the imagination into what that experience would be like.

I know a family who had two sons, fairly close in age. The two were in their early teens, and were out hunting together. One of them tripped, the shotgun went off, and it removed the back half of the other kid's head. What must it be like as the kid who accidently shot his brother? That moment will haunt him every minute of every day for the rest of his life. What must that be like for the parents who have both lost a child to a violent accident, and also are the parents of a child who killed another child in an accident? They catch both sides of that tragedy.

### "It Could Never Happen to Me"

We hear stories on the news about the craziest of things happening to people, like the baby in the hot car, or the accidental shooting among children. We shake our head as we can't begin to imagine dealing with something like that ourselves. We, as people, have a built-in mechanism that allows us to say, "That could never happen to me." We see horrible things happen to people, but basically go through our lives without generally fearing those exact circumstances. If we did fear every possible tragic circumstance, we would be frozen in place at all times.

I have not been in the military. I have never been in a combat zone, or in a third-world country. There are those who have, and who have seen things far more tragic, violent, horrifying, and gut-wrenching than me. The things I have dealt with are probably quite tame compared to things our soldiers see in other countries. So, there, I have acknowledged that fact. I don't want to be misleading, as if I believe I see the worst there is to see. I know I do not.

But, with that disclaimer out of the way, in the sense of the average non-military American, we see the worst that happens to people. There is no monitoring system at the door where we can turn ER cases away because they are too scary, or gross, or upsetting. Firefighters and EMT's are not made guarantees that they will never have to see something on the side of the highway that gives them nightmares for the remainder of their life. There are no promises that you will never do CPR on a tiny baby while the screaming mother watches. There are no promises that you will avoid seeing violently-deceased children. There are no promises that you can somehow avoid things that bother you. If it happens, and there is any chance of a life being saved, it will come into the ER. Nobody will ever stop you in the hall and warn you to brace yourself for what you are about to see. A charge nurse is never going to call you and ask if you are okay taking a certain kind of patient.

When I first was becoming a volunteer firefighter, even before I started my EMT training, I recall having a great deal of stress about the things I might see. I had this hope that I could go on calls to fires, and never have to see a burned person, and go to car wrecks and never see a mangled or dead person. I hoped that I would never have to see a decapitated head on the side of the highway, or brains having been violently removed from a person. I hoped that I would never respond to a motorcycle wreck and see broken leg bones sticking out through the skin. But there are no guarantees in this line of work. I saw some things, and didn't see other things. Had I stayed in that line of work long enough, I would have seen it all. But instead, I got into nursing, and so I saw a whole different set of horrors instead.

Most people out there see tragedies on the news, are moved by the horror of the story, and unconsciously believe, "It could never happen to me." And most of them would be right. Further, not only would most of them never experience a tragedy of that magnitude, but they would never even know a friend or family member who did. They have two degrees of removal from the situation. It was not them, and it was not anyone they know. This is a comforting fact for most people.

However, when you choose to work in the ER or ICU, or many other places in nursing, you will be part of those situations. Those things on the news that are so unimaginably horrifying that a normal person can only cope by quickly changing the channel and believing, "It could never happen to me..."

Well, you are the person who will see and experience those things. Those are the things that will be brought into your ER and ICU. You don't have the luxury of ignorance. You have chosen to stare tragedy right in the face, fight it, absorb it, and allow it to become a part of you as you work to save a life. That is a heroic calling. Not everybody can do it. There are many nurses who can't do it. And there are plenty of places for them to work, where they will not be exposed to this sort of thing.

You may choose a path that will put these horrors in front of you. But why would anybody want to expose themselves to that sort of thing? I don't think any of us like it, enjoy it, or desire to see it. But since it happens to people out there, we are called to stand by their side and fight for them. And we can take comfort knowing that if one day "it happens to me," a nurse will be there with us too.

# Chapter 16:   Final Thoughts

As I have said before, I love being a nurse, and could not picture myself doing anything different.  It is a fulfilling line of work, but also continuously challenges the nurse to learn new things, develop new skills, and gain expertise.  The job never settled into a cruise-control setting where there was nothing more to learn.

The complexities of the job seem to continuously increase, but the technology that support's the nurse's efforts keeps pace.  There was a time not long ago, when everything was done on paper.  The nurse and other administrative staff spent a great deal of time reviewing, processing, communicating, and then carrying out orders.  Medication orders on paper had to be approved by the nurse, and then faxed to the pharmacy for the medication to be filled.  Lab orders had to be sent to the lab in the same fashion, in order for a phlebotomist to show up.  Lab results were eventually brought to the unit printed on paper, when there was no computer system, and the massive amounts of notes, orders, documents, results, etc had to be managed on paper.  It was a full-time position for a unit clerk to complete these otherwise seemingly simple tasks, while the physicians and nurses continued to make changes in every way possible.  But the tasks were genuinely not simple, and larger units often required multiple unit clerks to keep up with the work flow.  It became a position requiring skill, expertise, multitasking, and the ability to think and work on the fly.

Nurses spent a great deal of time hand-writing notes and other documentation on paper.  The handwriting of physicians is notoriously and famously bad, leading to the ever-present threat of misunderstanding or mistake, leading to more interruptions, pages, phone calls, and written clarification orders. The paper chart was a cumbersome tool in the healthcare process.

Meanwhile, the life-support machines, testing equipment, medications, treatments, tools, devices, gadgets, knick-knacks, and gizmos have become more powerful, but also more challenging to master. The protocols and procedures endlessly grow in complexity, and it seems a new task in the normal workflow is added daily. Perhaps it's an extra bit of documentation now required on every patient, or a new way to screen every patient for a certain infection, or a new set of questions each patient must be asked.

At one point in one of my hospitals, we were suddenly required to obtain an anal swab on every single patient admitted to the hospital, to screen for a particular intestinal antibiotic-resistant bacteria that had become prominent in the region.

Me: "I need to swab your anus to check for an infection."

Patient: "But I am only here to be monitored overnight because my blood pressure was a little high."

Me: "Yes, now please present your anus for swabbing."

The requirements and processes for transporting patients off the unit for testing or procedures begins to involve more people, more phone calls, more paperwork, and greater monitoring. Practically all patients in every unit are on portable heart monitors now. That used to be reserved for patients with heart problems. The nurses must spend much more time printing, labeling, documenting, assessing, interpreting, uploading, and communicating EKG rhythm strips.

Sometimes it feels like there are people in suits in some office in another building who are just working to come up with more ways to complicate the nurse's life. Each day they strive to make another process more complex, by adding a new set of steps, checks, reviews, audits, and reports. There are always good intentions when coming up with new processes. In reality, they are done to fill a need, fix or prevent an occurring problem, or respond to a new law or regulation.

Through oversight organizations, hospitals have new requirements and restrictions placed on them, much of which directly affects the compensation they receive from Medicare, Medicaid, and insurance companies. As always, the following is a dynamic process that is changing over time, so my personal experience may be slightly dated... but... One major example recently was the monitoring of hospital "readmissions." If a patient was in the hospital for any reason, and then was admitted back to the hospital within a period of time, the hospital was financially penalized. No matter what the prior hospitalization was for, if the patient was readmitted with any one of a specific list of diagnoses, it was bad.

A major problem were things like chronic heart failure. If the patient is not compliant with their medications, diet, and fluid restrictions, they will get sick and be hospitalized. And it often happened, that a heart failure patient would be noncompliant, and have a readmission, and the hospital was penalized for the patient's failures, as if the hospital could control what the patient did at home. Major efforts were made to team with the local fire departments and EMS companies to do home visits to recently discharged patients with certain disease processes to monitor for compliance. You can see how the trajectory of something like that seems unsustainable.

But with the growing complexity comes tools and resources that help keep it flowing. Electronic health record systems are now universally in use, and vary in many ways in their function and complexity. As mentioned earlier in the book, it requires armies of computer people and medical

232

people to design and implement these systems, but then many chores and processes become streamlined and steps are eliminated. The productivity of the medical staff becomes more efficient. Physicians enter orders straight into the computer, essentially eliminating the need for a unit clerk. Since they enter the orders, the nurse is not caught in the middle trying to decide what a scribble means. The pharmacy automatically receives their orders, as does the lab, radiology, dietary, case management, therapists, and even clergy.

It can all be challenging for the older generation of nurses who had not previously used computers for anything. But the modern generation of nurses have grown up in a society that is tech-heavy. So computers are not intimidating and the learning curve for programs and changes is easier. In fact, in the rare occasion the system was "down" for a short period of time, for whatever reason, the nursing staff in the ICU would get into a panic, as they were trying to figure out how to write and process orders, and do documentation on paper.

Nursing is not for the stagnant-minded. It is different today than it was yesterday. And it will be different tomorrow than it is today. Nurses must be prepared to constantly learn and grow. Adaptability and flexibility are absolutely essential traits a nurse must have. And those traits must be supported by patience, willingness, and a healthy work ethic.

It is likely that the medical expertise of the nurse will continue on an upward trajectory. As there are emerging shortages of medical providers like family practice or primary care physicians, nurse practitioners will be taking on a more substantial role in managing the routine care of the population. In the current healthcare system I use for myself, I have actually never seen a physician for the routine primary-care stuff... Check blood pressure, get labs to check cholesterol again, change the dose on a blood pressure medication, address a sore throat, etc. These things can all be done by nurse practitioners and physician's assistants.

Nursing is an exciting field that will continue to grow and thrive for decades to come. Those entering the profession are correct to be excited about the work they will do, and inspired about the difference they will make. And while there are many things that keep changing, a few things always stay the same. One fixture in this realm is that nursing is not a job. It is an actual change in you as a person. You are not just a nurse in the hospital. You are still a nurse when you see somebody fall in the grocery store, or you drive by a car accident. You are still a nurse when you are out in a social setting, and your character is on display for the world. Are you behaving in a way that reflects appropriately on your profession? If one of your patients saw you in a club, or bar, or at a party, or a sporting event, would you be acting in a way that would disappoint them? Being identified as a nurse brings with it heightened expectations about personal conduct, trustworthiness, reverence for the human condition, and compassion for the fellow man.

I believe your character and integrity is not defined by how you act in front of people, but how you act when nobody is looking. Is your character and integrity, as a nurse, appropriate when you are alone? Can you be trusted to follow through with medications, treatments, vital signs, and documentation when the patient is unconscious and nobody is around to watch? Your patients are among the most vulnerable populations in the world. You have access to them, their private information, their secrets, their belongings, their families, and sometimes their homes. If you are a home health nurse, and the family leaves for the day, can they trust you to not steal something, or eat their food, or ignore their child? Will you cut corners because no one is looking? Will you document a task, when you actually never performed it? Will you "copy-and-paste" your daily assessments, instead of performing a new and thorough assessment each shift?

Consider an extreme example in which a nurse is caught up in a lie or is shown to have been derelict in their duties. A nurse is coming on shift, and she has received her assignment but has not gotten report from the prior nurse as the prior nurse is busy. So she decides to get a jump on vital signs and assessments. She runs into the first room where she is assigned, knocks out the process and is happy to have a head start as she's gotten that first one finished. She finds the off-going nurse at the nurse station and they begin report. The prior nurse pulls up the patient documentation to review and discuss, and sees the newly charted vital signs and head-to-toe assessments freshly entered by the oncoming nurse. The vital signs are nice and stable, and are consistent with those of the prior shift. The head-to-toe assessment virtually matches everything from the previous shifts, so we know the patient is stable and nothing is changing. Everything looks great!

The only problem is that the patient had died suddenly an hour earlier, and the family had already left, and a funeral home was expected any time to pick up the body. Had she waited for report, she would have learned the patient's disposition. But, now, she has officially charted a healthy blood pressure, heart rate, respiratory rate, and temperature, along with having heard normal heart and lung sounds, found appropriate pulses in the wrists and feet, having noted that the patient is appropriately alert (awake) and oriented (not confused), and that the patient has otherwise presented appropriate physical and neurological assessment results. Everything looks exactly like it did 12 hours prior, when the patient was in great shape.

The problem is clear. The nurse ran in the room and basically copied or fabricated every piece of assessment data from that of the previous shift. It can be done easily. When charting in the computer, you can easily see what the last ten entries were for a piece of information. This is helpful to know whether your findings are consistent with earlier findings, or if something is changing. But it can also present problematic temptations. For days, everyone had charted the pulses in the feet were located and appropriate. So, it's easy enough to just assume that trend has continued, and "copy-and-paste" the information. It saves precious time and energy as the nurse is stretched so thin. But have those pulses changed over time, and nobody has noticed because everybody stopped genuinely assessing?

But... the patient is really dead, and not a single piece of data the nurse has charted can possibly be true. What is her explanation? "Oh, I got confused?" "Oh, I think I charted on the wrong patient?" (Even though the assessment data and vitals match that exact patient). "Oh, I was practicing something with the charting system?" Is there really any reason the nurse can produce that will explain this away and cause no further question or concern?

This nurse has likely just lost her job, and will probably be dragged before a nursing review board, in which a panel of her peer nurses will examine the data, question her, and debate the circumstances of the situation. It's like being on trial. She will have an opportunity to explain herself, but will most likely be found as having been incompetent in her actions. She will be reported to the state board of nursing, who will open their own investigation, and she will either lose her license, or have it suspended.

Or, maybe the off-going nurse realizes what happened, and wants to cover for her friend, so they erase the information (or note that it was an entry error), and start over. Now, is the off-going nurse equally as guilty? Yes. Was anybody technically hurt? No. But, can we ever trust either nurse again? No. Do you, reader, want either of these nurses caring for your parents? No.

I have never seen anything quite this dramatic play out, but I have seen nurses fail to document assessment data or vitals for a shift, and the patient ends up dying. The nurse probably did nothing wrong in care and did not cause the death, but their lack of documentation puts the target on them when the doctor wants to blame somebody and deflect attention from his own decisions and orders. (We say "CYA" or "Cover Your Ass" in charting).

I have seen a CNA report blood sugar readings to the nurse that were fabricated. When the nurse was concerned that a reading did not align with her expectations (considering recent medications, etc), she rechecked the reading herself and got a totally different number. Upon reviewing the log in the glucometer device, there had been no blood sugar tests even done in recent hours, and certainly none of the results the CNA provided were present. Nurses dose insulin based on these numbers. That's an easy way to kill a patient.

Consider what it must be like to be the parent of a special needs child, especially one who is unable to speak or provide you with feedback on the nurses. If you have home health nursing, then you have a person, often a stranger, in your home day and night. You have no choice but to trust them, unless you want to go for days without sleep and not leave the child's side. Sure, after a while the nurse becomes well known, familiar, and almost like part of the family. But in most cases, nurses are always turning over and changing. How would you feel if every day you had a new stranger show up at your door, and you had to grant them full access to your vulnerable child, and had to grant full access to your home? And, this stranger will be left alone with your child and in your home while you are away during the day, or up in your home all night while you sleep.

Maybe you learn that this was the nurse who

fabricated the assessment from earlier.  She got fired from her job, but salvaged her license.  Now, she works in home health, and is your home.  Can you trust her?  Would you ever trust her?  Is there a statement of contrition or act of penance sufficient enough to "clear the slate" and grant the nurse blind trust again?

It takes a lifetime to earn true and genuine trust.  But it only takes one instant or one event to destroy it all.  But we, as nurses, do not have a lifetime to earn the trust that is put in us.  We just have a few years of school and a few years of a clean employment record.  The responsibility lies with us to self-manage, to be honest with ourselves, to hold ourselves accountable.  If I would not do something in front of people, but I would be willing to do it when no one is looking, can I even trust myself?

Nurses are among the most trusted professions in the world.  I have a story I like to use from my experience.  I was working in the ER, and was assigned to the desk in the waiting room, where I would check people in and monitor those waiting.  The door opened and a young mother ran as fast as she could toward me.  She was cradling a tiny baby, and she was screaming that her baby was not breathing.  As I saw her coming, I stood and began pushing everything out of the way where I could lay the baby down on my desk and start CPR.  As the woman neared my desk, she reached out and forcefully thrust the baby into my arms.

It was a moment of clear and unfiltered panic for her.  But I was there.  I was in scrubs.  I had a stethoscope around my neck.  I had a badge that said "nurse."

The woman did not know my name.  She did not stop to ask where I went to school or what my grades were.  She did not ask to see my employee reviews, or get references from my bosses and coworkers.  She did not ask how long I had been a nurse.  She did not know if I was a good or bad person, friendly or rude, new or experienced, well-rested or

238

tired, whether I had a nice family at home or had my own tragedies. She didn't even know what language I might have spoken as I never had a chance to speak.

But, I was there, in medical scrubs, with a stethoscope around my neck, and a badge that said "nurse." So, she thrust her tiny baby into my arms, entrusting me with this tiny life that she loved more than anything in the world. I like to reflect on that moment occasionally. There were hundreds or maybe thousands of other moments over the years that rival that situation. There was probably a situation every single day that was at least this meaningful. But this particular case has just always stuck with me.

You're not a person working as a nurse. You are a nurse. You are the job. You are the profession, the trust, and the dignity that comes with it. And you maintain this identity 24 hours a day, and seven days a week. As I have disclosed, I am not currently working, and have not for a couple of years. I do not know if I will again. I hope so. But, in the meantime, even though I am not currently employed and actively "doing the job," I still consider myself a nurse, and I always will. If I never work again, I will still be a nurse. It's who I am, it's who I will always be. The knowledge, skill, experiences, memories, lessons learned, lives touched... They are all part of me, and will be always, no matter what.

So, since I have kept you in suspense. To answer your question, yes, the baby survived. Upon taking the baby from the mother and having a split second to assess as I was placing it on the desk to start CPR, I found that it was indeed breathing. Its breathing was fast, shallow, and sounded terrible. It was clearly very sick, and was going to be in serious trouble if medical care was not provided soon. But it was breathing. No CPR was needed. I assured the mother we were going to take care of everything, and quickly carried the baby back to a triage room to hand off to another nurse, as the mother followed.

Brett Craigsly

Again, this single moment and situation that unfolded over the course of less than 60 seconds included dramatic concepts of life-and-death, fear, panic, loss, grief, trust, surrender... How many people out there in the world have had a newborn baby thrust into their arms during a medical emergency? A single incident as dramatic and intense as this one might come along once in a lifetime for a non-medical person, or maybe never at all. The other people in the waiting room all watched it unfold with wide eyes and looks of fear, panic, and concern. They were afraid they were about to watch me do CPR on a baby that might be dead.

But there I was, scrubs, stethoscope, badge, clocked-in for work, at my assigned duty station, doing my routine job. My heart rate did not elevate during that event, nor did I experience an adrenalin rush. I did not panic, or even get nervous. I knew what to do. Because I am a nurse.

And perhaps the most interesting part of the story is what followed. After handing off the baby and mother to the triage nurse, I quietly returned to my desk and sat down. As I sat and looked around, I noted that all eyes in the waiting room were on me. The looks of concern and fear continued as the other waiting patients whispered to each other about what they just witnessed. (Not me being a hero. But whispering about the medical scare of a possibly dying baby) I just gave a half-smile and friendly nod to the room and resumed my paperwork.

This is the job we have. When we complete the task, we go right back to work. The same thing might happen 20 more times that day, or maybe something even crazier. Maybe we would do CPR multiple times as patients were being unloaded from helicopters on the roof or in the parking lot. Maybe we would see an unspeakable horror as a trauma victim is brought in with body parts missing. Maybe we would hold the hand of a dying patient and minister to the grieving family. Maybe we would physically wrestle with a

240

violent psychiatric patient, or have to sit in a room to monitor a suicidal patient. Maybe we would care for a child who had been abused... physically, sexually, emotionally... Maybe we would work with a battered wife as she tries to escape her abusive home. Maybe we would take care of a car wreck patient, who knows that their friend or family member did not survive. Or maybe the wreck was the fault of that patient, and they know they have killed others by accident. Maybe we will take care of a dying gunshot victim, and as we work to save their life, we are following procedures to preserve evidence, and we are surrounded by detectives who will be working to solve the murder. Or... maybe it would all be twisted ankles and sore throats that day.

This one situation with the baby was just one of thousands of situations I saw in my career. I have thousands of stories. I have seen the wildest of things. I have seen the worst tragedies and have had a front-row seat to watch genuine human suffering, but I have also witnessed miracles. I have seen joy and hope and peace amidst the most dire of circumstances. I have seen the best and the worst humanity has to offer.

Whatever the case, we are there, in our scrubs, with a stethoscope around our neck, a badge that says 'nurse," and we are ready for anything. That is all anybody needs to know about us. The resulting trust is automatic. It's an exciting life. And at the end of the day, as humble heroes always say, "don't thank me, I'm just doing my job."

I hope I have been able to provide some knowledge, some laughs, and a little inspiration to those who are in pursuit of a life as a nurse. I don't know everything, but I'm hoping my story might be a guide to assist others in their journey.

If you have the right spirit, nursing is an adventure, and both exciting and fulfilling. It certainly was for me. I hope it will be for you too. God Bless!

241

**Check out Brett Craigsly's other recently-released titles on Amazon and Kindle!**

A harrowing tale of one nurse's struggles with addiction, deceit, and crime. However, facing his demons proves difficult when he must question what is real and what is only in his mind. Nurse Brady faces danger from every direction, including from within, as he struggles to define himself. Is he good? Is he evil? Maybe both. Perhaps he is his own worst demon. But in the meantime, can he even survive the world in which he exists as the threats pile up? This thoughtful drama builds into a thrilling action story, and keeps the reader always guessing.

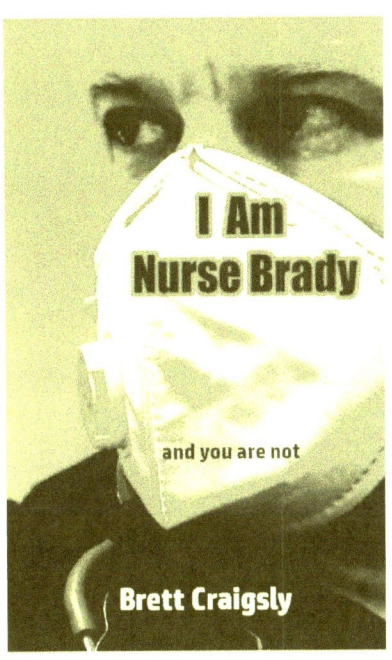

Meet four strangers who find themselves locked in a psychiatric unit alone. With no doctors or nurses, the insanity is in charge. They must fight to escape, but first they must fight for their lives. Is there a dark force at work? Or are they victims of their own minds?

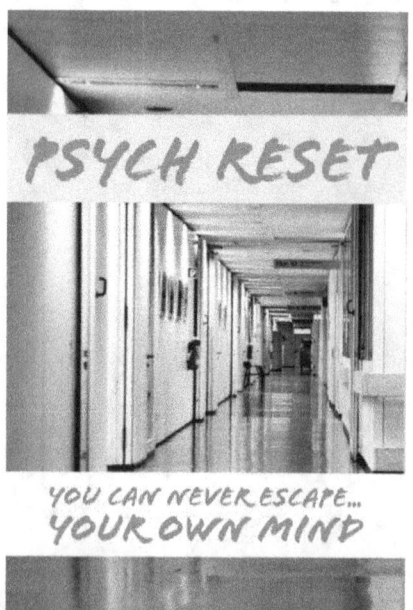

PSYCH RESET

YOU CAN NEVER ESCAPE...
YOUR OWN MIND

BRETT CRAIGSLY

Parking Lot Lamentations is the uncomfortable image we see when we look in the mirror and really begin to ask questions. Many would probably rather not think about such things. It might threaten their peace about their place in the world. With knowledge and enlightenment comes hardship. Ignorance, naivety, and oblivion can be blissful.

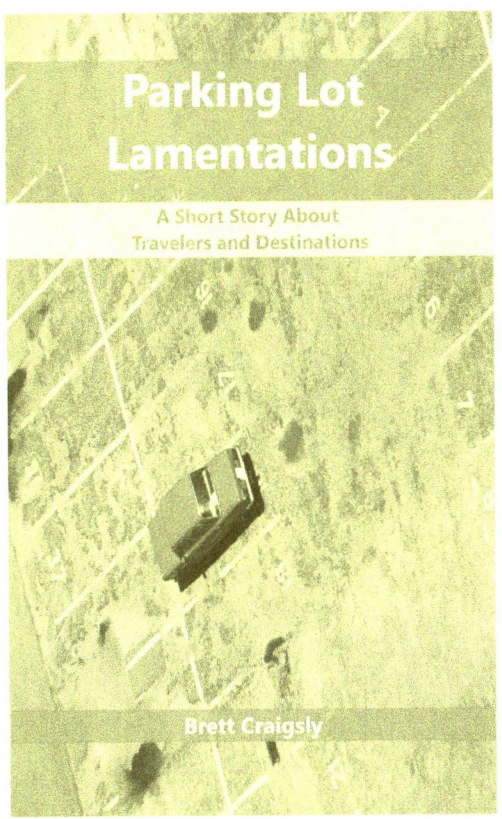